LEAN ON ME

TEN POWERFUL STEPS TO

MOVING BEYOND YOUR

DIAGNOSIS AND TAKING

BACK YOUR LIFE

Nancy Davis

A FIRESIDE BOOK
Published by Simon & Schuster
New York   London   Toronto   Sydney

"Lean on Me" by Bill Withers © 1972, renewed 2000 by Interior Music Corp. All rights administered by Songs of Universal, Inc./BMI. Used by permission. All Rights Reserved.

FIRESIDE
Rockefeller Center
1230 Avenue of the Americas
New York, NY 10020

Designed by Katy Riegel

Manufactured in the United States of America

1 3 5 7 9 10 8 6 4 2

Library of Congress Cataloging-in-Publication Data is available

ISBN-13: 978-0-7432-7640-5
ISBN-10: 0-7432-7640-X

For information regarding special discounts for bulk purchases,
please contact Simon & Schuster Special Sales at
1-800-456-6798 or business@simonandschuster.com.

DEDICATION

This book is dedicated to Marvin and Barbara Davis, my father and mother, who passionately instilled in me the true value of charity and the importance of never taking "No" for an answer when it comes to your health.

This book is also dedicated to my patient and loving husband, Kenny, and my five precious children—Brandon, Alexander, Jason, Isabella, and Mariella. My family is the real reason that I fought to regain my health and will fight to stay healthy in the future. I want to celebrate and enjoy the privilege of being a happy wife and mother every day. I love my family from the deepest part of my heart.

Lean on Me

Sometimes in our lives we all have pain
We all have sorrow
But if we are wise
We know that there's always tomorrow

Lean on me, when you're not strong
And I'll be your friend
I'll help you carry on
For it won't be long
'Til I'm gonna need
Somebody to lean on

Please swallow your pride
If I have things you need to borrow
For no one can fill those of your needs
That you don't let show

Lean on me, when you're not strong
And I'll be your friend
I'll help you carry on
For it won't be long
'Til I'm gonna need
Somebody to lean on

If there is a load you have to bear
That you can't carry
I'm right up the road
I'll share your load
If you just call me

So just call on me brother, when you need a hand
We all need somebody to lean on
I just might have a problem that you'd understand
We all need somebody to lean on

Lean on me when you're not strong
And I'll be your friend
I'll help you carry on
For it won't be long
Till I'm gonna need
Somebody to lean on

CONTENTS

HOW TO USE
THIS BOOK

It would be wonderful if this book was given as a graduation gift for every high school or college student. It contains important information that everyone will need at some point in life. We all need to understand the fundamentals of taking responsibility for our own lives and our own health, but there are few classes taught in school that provide this basic knowledge. Realistically, when you find yourself or a friend in a life-altering situation, you will want to read this book as soon as possible.

You have come into possession of this book because either you or someone you love is already facing a major medical crisis. You may need help in a specific area. Most likely, that area is covered by one or more of the ten steps I have outlined in this book. Although I learned the lessons of these steps in approximately the same order as I have presented them, you may need to start immediately on a particular section, develop your understanding from there, then come back to the other chapters later as different crises present themselves.

For example, if you are in a hospital emergency room and are fortunate enough to have this book in your hands, read the short section "ER Basics" at the back of this book. You may not have prepared for the emergency room visit, but the information provided will teach you quickly how to stay in control of the situation, how to help the ER personnel, and how to understand what is going on around you.

If your doctor has given you a copy of this book because you have just been diagnosed, please go home, sit down quietly, and read my introduction, "You're Lucky." I believe that it will be a comfort and an inspiration for you. I have been where you are now, and I know that you are going through many of the difficult emotions and experiences I describe. You must turn hopelessness into hopefulness. I am absolutely sincere about the title of this book: *Lean on Me*. If you or your loved one or friend suddenly finds his or her life turned upside down with a devastating illness, you will understand the importance of the phrase, "We all need somebody to lean on."

Perhaps you are a relative or a close friend of someone who has just been diagnosed with a devastating illness. First, put a copy of this book into this person's hands. If reading is difficult, offer to read it to him or her. Second, skim the entire contents and see what seems to apply to the most pressing problem that you or your friend or relative is facing. Absorb that section and take appropriate action.

Undoubtedly there will be many people who have heard that I have useful advice about how to deal with the medical establishment. You need this help especially if you feel that you do not have the insurance or financial ability to get the health care you need. Remember that no matter what your current financial situation, you have the right to the best care possible.

Please turn to Step Nine, "Tame the Health Care Monster," to see if I have addressed your specific problems. The information in the resources section will take you further.

If your parent has chronic medical problems, you may have obtained this book as a guide to advocacy. Consider this a fresh start, a new way of looking at your parent's problems. This is the time when you may have to reverse roles and become your parent's caretaker, just as he or she has always cared for you. There are a variety of positive elements to be introduced as you implement the ten steps. You will definitely see how these concepts apply to your life, too.

Finally, if you are that rare and truly lucky person who is not facing an immediate medical crisis in your life or in a loved one's life, I hope this book will inspire you to take charge of your life and prepare intelligently for a medical crisis that surely will affect you or a loved one in the future. I hope these steps will give you the strength and independence that they have given me. I hope my story will empower you and encourage you to live your life in a way that will inspire and help others.

INTRODUCTION

"You're Lucky"

FOURTEEN YEARS AGO, when I was first diagnosed with a degenerative and life-threatening disease, the last thing in the world I wanted to hear was someone telling me that I was lucky. I did not feel lucky. I felt my life unraveling before my very eyes.

The nightmare began while I was on a ski vacation in Aspen. At the time I was a thirty-three-year-old wife and mother of three precious sons, soaking up the vibrations of the Rocky Mountain slopes, which I had loved since junior high school. Having moved to Los Angeles with my family a few years earlier, being back in the familiar terrain of my youth was like coming home.

I was euphoric, and I went overboard—taking nonstop ski runs one after another, pushing myself to go ever faster. Never mind the poor visibility and the dangerous patches of blue ice spotting the snow pack. Never mind that everybody had quit for the day because the conditions were so bad. It was the last day of a ten-day Christmas vacation, and I had never skied so well. My head was full and I just had to keep going for the last run of the day.

I get a knot in my stomach every time I think of that day. No matter what the risk, I was determined to do it. I rationalized the danger by telling myself that I needed this last bit of exercise, that if I burned a few more calories, pushed myself just a bit harder, I would feel better and look thinner. I was trying to recapture my reckless youth, and I was feeling much more confident in my athletic abilities than I should have.

In retrospect, I understand that muscle tone and thrill-seeking were not my only motivations. I was in a desperate race to run from myself, to escape nagging thoughts about my deteriorating marriage. Racing headlong down a mountain slope with the wind in your face, poised to throw yourself into a hairpin turn in a fraction of a second, doesn't give you a chance to reflect on where you've been, or where you are emotionally.

My instincts were telling me not to take the extra run, but I was not listening. I had turned that part of myself off quite some time ago. The next thing I knew I was losing my balance. I slid across an unseen patch of ice on one ski. Propelled forward by my own momentum, I was totally out of control. The last thing I remember thinking was, Why did my bindings fail to release? Finally, I heard a disturbing *pop* in my knee, and every nerve in my body screamed out in excruciating pain.

LISTEN TO YOUR BODY

By now you may be wondering what my ski accident possibly has to do with my contracting a debilitating disease. A person doesn't get diabetes, arthritis, cancer, Parkinson's, multiple sclerosis, or AIDS from skiing in the Rockies, surfing in Malibu, or bungee jumping in Hawaii. It took me nearly a full decade and a major paradigm shift in my thinking to understand the subtle connections that link disease, lifestyle, and the mental conditioning that brings on illness. I might not have been skiing at all had I not been in such a rush to escape the unpleasant reality of my marriage. And I may not have lost my balance on the ski slope that day if my immune system had not become overactive and had begun to attack the myelin of my central nervous system. Had I stopped to listen to what my body was so desperately trying to tell me, I might have avoided the nightmare to come. At the very least, I would have viewed what happened to me as a wake-up call and not a death sentence.

The emergency room doctor at the Aspen Valley Hospital evaluated me and diagnosed my injury. I'd torn a ligament, the anterior cruciate ligament (ACL), in my right knee. Not that it was any big deal—at the time this was considered the Aspen equivalent of the common cold. I was fitted with a brace, set up with a course of physical therapy, and sent back to Los Angeles the following day. After seeking several second opinions, I was scheduled to return to Aspen for an operation to be performed by Dr. Mark Purnell, one of the most skillful knee surgeons in the country.

SYMPTOMS BEGIN TO APPEAR

Three weeks to the day after tearing my ACL, but before the surgery, I woke up to find that I had lost all feeling in the tips of my three middle fingers of my right hand. I shook them, thinking that I must have slept in an awkward position, that my fingers were simply "asleep." The problem was that they would not wake up. Maybe the torn ligament or the knee brace was too tight, or maybe it was those electrodes they placed all over me during physical therapy. Three days later I lost all feeling in my

entire right hand. This time I called an orthopedist in Los Angeles to find out how all this was connected. It was not connected to my knee injury, he said, and recommended I see a
neurologist.

A neurologist? My first thought was that the orthopedist was
covering up for something he had done wrong. I was not going
to call. The numbness would go away. Besides, I did not have
time to see another doctor. I was going to be fine. Doctors were
for sick people, little children, and the elderly, not a young
mother with three active boys, ages six, eight, and ten.

Three days later, I woke up without any feeling in the finger-
tips of the three middle fingers of my other hand. Like clock-
work, another three days passed and there was no feeling in
either hand. Immediately, I made an appointment with the
neurologist. By the time I arrived in his office, I had also lost all
feeling in my stomach. My eyesight was starting to blur. I had
mild flu symptoms as well.

Now I was really worried. I was more than ready to overcome my previous resistance to seeing another doctor. I just
wanted someone to explain why this very peculiar paralysis was
spreading throughout my body in such a systematic way, what
was going to happen next, and how soon they could fix whatever was wrong with me so I could get on with my life.

THE MRI

Not soon enough, apparently. It was Friday afternoon. The
neurologist did some general tests and a blood workup and told
me I needed more tests. He ordered an MRI for Sunday, an indication that whatever was going on was serious enough to warrant immediate attention. "Don't worry," he said. "The MRI
will only last three hours." It occurred to me that any X-ray
technician working on a Sunday might not be the best the de-

partment had to offer, but once again I ignored the voice in the back of my mind issuing me a warning.

At dinner that night, after my three sons, Brandon, Alexander, and Jason, had left the table unaware of the symptoms I was having, I casually mentioned the MRI to my husband. I didn't want to make a big deal out of something I was still thinking was a fluke complication related to my skiing accident. True to form, he was angry at me for putting a damper on *his* weekend. "Can't you just go on Monday? Sunday is *my* day," he declared. "I'm busy. You can take care of it."

"Can you help with the boys while I'm there?"

"No. I told you: I have my own plans. Don't ruin my weekend. You only think of yourself," he said. Subject closed.

On Sunday, three of my dearest girlfriends—Lynn Palmer, Brenda Richie, and Kathryn Belton—insisted on taking me to the MRI appointment, putting their obligations and their families' plans aside to be with me for what turned into eight interminable hours.

"Hold still," the technician repeated every time I coughed or moved, which was quite frequent. In addition to all my other symptoms, I had the flu. He scanned the same parts of my body over and over again as I lay on the gurney feeling ready to explode with frustration. My conclusion was that he had to be the most incompetent X-ray technician in all of Los Angeles. Why was he the only one working on a Sunday? He must be in training, I thought.

Meanwhile, I joked with my friends to hide my impatience and nervousness, as the promised three hours turned into seven. Lynn, my confidante, who is often mistaken for my sister, seemed to be nervous and fighting back tears. I couldn't understand why she was acting as she did, instead of being her usual peppy and fun self. Brenda and Kathryn were uncharacteristically quiet and sat stiffly, blank expressions on their faces. Later,

I learned that even though he had not said anything to me, the unthinking technician had told my friends that the MRI showed spots on my brain and spinal column—which could have been any number of things, none of them good. I had to wait for my appointment with the neurologist to hear the news the next day, but the tone and tenor of what I was about to be told had already been set into motion without my knowing it. My normally fun-loving friends drove me home in an eerie silence, looking at me strangely.

THE DIAGNOSIS

Twenty-four hours later I was in the neurologist's office. My mother had come with me, but after more than an hour in the waiting room, I urged her to go home, assuring her that there was nothing to worry about. The minute they called my name, however, I profoundly regretted that she wasn't by my side.

Inside the inner sanctum of the doctor's office, a bright light was streaming through the MRIs of my brain and spinal column. They spread over the doctor's walls like blotchy wallpaper. The neurologist reminded me of Darth Vader as he held out a long high-tech laser pointer, indicating various spots on the surreal images. He seemed to be performing a ritual dance, one he had performed countless times before for other sick patients. The real problem was that although Nancy Davis was the name on the MRIs, there was obviously some mistake: he couldn't possibly be talking about me.

"You see this spot on your brain?" Dr. Vader pointed to the MRI. "See this one . . . and this one . . . and this one."

I was having an out-of-body experience. I saw myself standing next to him, confused, staring at the incomprehensible display. That isn't my body, I said to myself. I am invincible! Nothing can be wrong with me. I am a mom to three precious boys who need my love, protection, guidance, and full-time energy and attention. I am way too busy and impossibly impatient. I don't do *sick*. It simply isn't in my job description. I'm not good at it. There is absolutely no time for this.

On the outside I looked like the same me: boundlessly energetic and athletic, a young woman fully engaged in life's great adventure. I certainly did not look like a person with spots on her spinal column and her brain. Of course, just what was that person supposed to look like?

Then again, who was I to argue with this doctor, this medical messiah who had come so highly recommended? And suddenly, with the realization of my powerlessness to contest his verdict, I crash landed back on earth, back into my body. The room started to spin and I reached for a nearby chair.

The doctor still had not given a name to whatever it was that was wrong with me. "Dear God," I prayed silently, "please make this something insignificant. Better still, make it a mistake, a common medical mix-up." After all, the X-ray technician could have mixed up the MRIs.

"And these spots on your spinal column," the neurologist continued, talking now in circles, "see this one, and this one." And then, "Wow, look how much bigger this area is!"

Finally, I couldn't take it any longer. Looking him square in the eyes, I asked point-blank what he was trying to tell me.

I gulped, swallowed, and mentally prepared to hear my fate—one that I sensed was going to change the course of my life as I knew it.

"You are very lucky," he said. "You have a disease called multiple sclerosis."

"Lucky?" I asked incredulously, sure that I had misheard his diagnosis.

"Oh, yes, you're lucky that you don't have a brain tumor. We were able to rule that out."

Lucky was the last thing I was feeling at that moment.

The doctor glanced at his watch. That gesture said so much:

it was late in the day, he had squeezed me into his schedule, and it was time to wrap it up.

PLEASE ANSWER MY QUESTIONS

But I still had questions. How do I fix it? I didn't know what to do. What was this going to mean for my quality of life, my independence, my future, and my children's future? The words *multiple sclerosis* conjured foggy images: people in wheelchairs, slouched over, unable to control their bodies. How soon was this going to happen to me? Did I have a choice?

I asked him to explain what MS really is. "It's a disease of the central nervous system," he said. "The word *multiple* means 'many,' and *sclerosis* means 'scars.' Thus, the term *multiple sclerosis* refers to the 'many scars' that form on the brain and spinal column in someone with the disease."

"How did I get it?" I asked. He shrugged, implying that it remained a medical mystery.

I pleaded, "Is there a cure? Is there medicine, surgery? What can I read? What do I do?" Illness had struck my family in the past, and I knew there were always options in the form of therapies and treatments.

"There is nothing you can do," the neurologist said. "Absolutely nothing." Then, adopting an expression that I imagined was supposed to pass for compassion, he concluded, "Go home and go to bed."

"For how long," I asked, "a few days, a week?"

He shook his head. "Go to bed . . . forever."

Again he reminded me that I was lucky: "You can have people bring food to you in bed," he said. Doing anything productive was out of the question; becoming a vegetable was my fate. As he walked to his door, he added thoughtfully, "You should be able to operate the remote control to your TV set."

He can't be serious, I thought, waiting for a clue that he had just made a tasteless joke. Only he was serious. Dead serious.

A flashback to my childhood and to the few times I was sick when my parents kept me home brought back memories of soap operas playing endlessly on the television, and bowls of cold, congealing chicken noodle soup. As much as I hated being sick, self-pity was far worse. I had to find something to do, an action that I could take. I was angry. How delusional could this doctor be to tell me that I was lucky?

"Do you have anything I can read about MS or that you might recommend I read?" I asked. There was nothing that he could recommend. I asked about ongoing research. Again his answer was not encouraging. Although there were some studies being done, none had produced meaningful results. "How about vitamins, special foods, something to take for the numbness?" I grasped.

The doctor was still standing in the doorway, holding the door open. Before I could finish, he cut me off. "Time to go," he said impatiently. "You know, rush hour. You don't want to get stuck in traffic, do you?"

MY EMOTIONAL DAM BURSTS

I exited his office dazed. Much of what the doctor had explained to me while looking at the MRIs sounded like a foreign language. The only thing I walked away with was a sense of dread. I left the office, as millions of other people do, not knowing what to do next. The greater tragedy is that most people who undergo this experience resign themselves to living a life of quiet desperation and never receiving answers to the important questions. They leave accepting the doctor's dire prognosis: no cure, no hope, and no life.

The numbness of my emotions now matched the lack of

physical sensation in my midsection and in my hands. As I hob-
bled toward the elevator, I became keenly aware of the pain in
my injured knee. The elevator doors opened and I stepped into
a space crowded with strangers—mostly professionals glad to be
leaving work for the day—and my emotional dam burst. I
looked at the faces of those strangers, and for the first time, perhaps since my early childhood, I appreciated the simple gift of
standing. I sobbed as the elevator began to descend. I gushed to
the point of hysteria, reaching an emotional place I had never
been before. The people watching me in the elevator were very
uncomfortable and flooded out of there the second the doors
opened. I suddenly felt jealous that they could all so easily walk
or run out of there and how easily their bodies functioned.

My first call before driving home was not to my husband but
to my mother. She was devastated, and she swung into action,
assuring me that she and my father would be at my house when
I got home. She also suggested that we get the neurologist on
the phone to answer all of our questions. "Drive carefully,"
Mom said. "Don't worry. Somehow we will figure this out," she
said in a very nervous voice.

It took me months, and then years, to understand fully that I
was indeed fortunate to still be alive: lucky to have my children, lucky for having understanding and supportive parents,
and lucky that as long as there was still breath in my lungs,
there was hope for everything.

Most important, I was a determined individual who did not
take no for an answer. MS or any other debilitating disease just
didn't fit in with my game plan. I couldn't imagine myself as a
hopeless vegetable. My inability to picture myself as an unfor-
tunate victim of circumstances beyond my control was, I believe, the determining factor in preventing me from becoming
just what the doctor had predicted. Acceptance of the physician's prognosis—no cure, no life, no hope—is a virus far more

deadly than anything a biologist can detect with a microscope. The prognosis you give yourself is the only one that is important. You can't allow yourself to accept a negative prognosis.

My early physical symptoms ran the MS gamut—numbness, tingling, extreme fatigue, vision problems, dizziness, and loss of motor control in my hands. There were times when I gave in to the common refrain: "This can't be happening to me! I don't deserve this! Poor me!" I experienced denial, shock, anger, blame, guilt, self-pity, and depression—all natural human reactions. I came to see that being diagnosed with a life-altering and possibly life-threatening disease is like experiencing the death of a loved one. I discovered that going through the roller coaster of emotional ups and downs is as crucial as grieving or mourning. I just did not get mired down in feeling sorry for myself. I would let myself feel the pain and conflicted emotions, and then I would move forward. I made a new game plan geared toward cultivating a positive attitude and finding readily accessible anchors to pull me through the rough times and help me appreciate the good times.

THE PROCESS OF SELF-EDUCATION

In the early days after my diagnosis, I learned that the way to find helpful information about the causes and treatments of an illness is riddled with roadblocks and misinformation. At the time, not much was known about MS, and what little information there was did not extend beyond the medical community. There were no therapies or drugs that could help stop the progression of MS. There were no uniform treatments that doctors prescribed. Every book I read led me nowhere. There were books on MS research studies, all of which ended up with negative results. At the time, it was next to impossible to find even basic answers to the many questions I had about this insidious, potentially disabling disease that was now going to be the label of my life. I did remember, however, hearing about people with terminal illnesses given six months to live, but finding strength, defying the odds, and still living ten to twenty years later.

The clock was ticking away. I would soon learn that the information void and misinformation maze are not unique to MS; they exist for most diseases that affect many hundreds of millions of people each year. As a result, I set out to educate myself in spite of the lack of information. I became a voracious consumer of anything and everything having to do with MS, my rather unpopular disease. I always had a battery of questions on hand for every doctor I spoke with. I approached friends and friends of friends. I was so thirsty for information and there was so little available to me that I even took to talking about my disease with strangers on planes and in restaurants.

I gradually began learning the things that I should have been told from the start. One of the theories about the genesis of MS is that people contract the disease in their midteens as a virus of which they are unaware. The autoimmune problem can lie dormant until the person is between the ages of twenty and forty. I learned that many people believe that one of three conditions brings on an MS attack: an illness, a physical injury, or extreme stress triggered by emotional trauma. At the time of my diagnosis, I was beset by all three—a torn ligament, the flu, and the ongoing trauma of my crumbling marriage.

I soon became totally consumed with making myself healthy and understanding the science of what was taking place in my body. There was always someone who could add some tidbit to my arsenal of knowledge. For what was then a relatively unknown disease, I was surprised at the number of people I encountered who knew someone who had been diagnosed with MS. To make the most of their advice, I had to learn not only how best to communicate but how to listen. I had to learn to make medicine understandable. It is not a mystery. The sophisticated Latin terms thrown out at you by doctors can all be translated into plain English and made totally understandable. Medicine does not require a rocket scientist to figure it out, however much most physicians communicate with one another in a completely foreign terminology. Make sure that your doctors take the time to explain your condition in language you can understand.

This is not a biology lesson. This is your one and only life.

BE YOUR OWN BEST ADVOCATE

I became my own best advocate in negotiating the labyrinth that our medical system has become. Then as today, the barriers were many: bureaucratic, corporate, and professional self-interest hinders a patient from obtaining the best treatments. The entire health care industry has become so powerful and disproportionately lucrative that it is now in the illness rather than the health business. By necessity I learned how to keep records of my visits to medical practitioners and specialists.

Learning to choose the best doctors to assist in my recovery proved to be more difficult than I had ever supposed. Paying top dollar to consult physicians with the best reputations does not guarantee success. The doctor who is right for someone else is not necessarily right for you.

The important thing to do is to trust your instincts. If something sounds wrong, if a physician or a treatment just does not work for you, if there is some detail about the procedure that bothers you, you have to listen very carefully to your body and educate yourself before moving forward. Don't ignore the little voice in the back of your head that issues warnings. Heed your instincts; understand why you may be feeling as you do. Learn everything you can about your disease, and then decide on a course of action. Trust yourself.

I didn't know, when I began my journey, that patients, too, have a bill of rights (see page 70), and that you do yourself a disservice by accepting anything less than the best a physician, medical practitioner, or hospital can give you. No subject is off limits for discussion. You have to become your own medical specialist and not be intimidated by doctors who are supposed to know more about you than you do. Ideally, no one should know more about you and your body than you do.

TAKE ACTION

I didn't just learn to "cope" with my deteriorating marriage and fear of how my medical condition would adversely affect my children. I did something about it. I surgically removed—in divorce court—the excess baggage of my miserable husband. I then set about building a new family dynamic in which my children, my parents, and my friends, along with physicians, therapists, and medical practitioners, became partners in my recovery rather than added emotional congestion. A large part of this process involved doing my own heavy lifting—just getting out of bed for starters. The important factor to remember is that you must stay engaged with life, even as you are being pressured to withdraw. I had to learn to celebrate the victories, no matter how large or small, and make a big deal about them.

The choices I made and the self-education I undertook allowed me to develop and stick to a health regimen that combined traditional and alternative therapies that were right for me. I learned to think of my body as the beautifully designed healing system that it is; to listen to what it was telling me and to act on that information rather than try to mask it or drive it underground. I ignored the traditional wisdom that a patient's state of mind does not matter to viruses and bacteria, and learned how and why it does. Fear can be as detrimental as overmedication. And just as the mind can invite illness into one's life, so can the mind be marshaled to repair the damage.

CHANGING NEGATIVES INTO POSITIVES

Now, in addition to getting plenty of exercise, eating healthful and nutritious foods, boosting my immune system with heavy doses of vitamins and nutritional supplements, and avoiding social and environmental conditions that invite illness, I incorporate prayer into my daily activities. I have learned to make my own mental MRIs that I can use to picture the physiological changes taking place in my body. Using these mental images has helped me, in many cases, to reverse what was taking place. Most physicians looked on what I was doing as a pointless exercise, yet the combined results were beyond anyone's expectations . . . except my own.

Today I am happier and healthier than I dreamed possible on the day I was first diagnosed. I have gone beyond just trying to heal myself; I have sought to raise the consciousness of the millions of people who have been or will be diagnosed with a life-changing disease. I have also raised millions of dollars for medical research and created a foundation that brings together teams of scientists and clinicians dedicated to developing innovative programs and therapeutic approaches to eradicate MS. It is the team approach that has helped me, and the team approach, which will, one day, remove MS and the other debilitating degenerative diseases from our vocabulary.

I have happily remarried and recently celebrated the birth of twin girls. I make frequent ski trips and I have a black belt in karate. I am able to do the very things that the doctors predicted I would never be able to do again.

The nightmare of being told "You're lucky" has taken on

unimagined meaning in my life. What had first seemed like a death sentence has turned out to be a blessing. In meeting the challenge of living with MS, I changed for the better. I became a much stronger, more evolved, and compassionate person. I tested myself in new ways. I took charge of my life.

I am not disease-free and might never be. I am not a doctor, a medical or psychological authority, or a self-help guru. I am someone who was given a devastating diagnosis and who sought practical ways to overcome my illness and live a full and meaningful life. I am now proud to call myself lucky. I am lucky to have my health.

The ten steps I describe in this book are practical measures designed to jump-start your healing process—no matter what life-altering or life-threatening disease you have. These are tools of health and self-preservation I wish I had known when I was first diagnosed. They invite you to face life's challenges, to imagine the possibilities beyond illness, to move beyond traditional limitations, and never to take no for an answer. The personal stories I have included, together with my own, are those of friends, colleagues, and acquaintances I've collected through my fourteen-year struggle with disease. These are the heroic stories of people with cancer, diabetes, muscular dystrophy, Parkinson's, AIDS, and other debilitating illnesses who have decided to defy the odds.

The diagnosis that you have been given is not a death sentence. It is an invitation to rebuild your life in a new and meaningful way. For people living with a debilitating disease, this message of hope can be as powerful as a cure. I know it was for me.

STEP ONE

Embrace Change

OUT OF EVERYTHING BAD comes something good. When something profoundly bad happens to you, it is very hard to see the light at the end of the tunnel. However, believe me that no matter how long it takes, you will emerge a very different person with amazing wisdom. You will see how this challenge has made your life more meaningful. MS has been the catalyst for profound change in my life. It gave me a complete career in an area I would never have imagined. It helped me to develop greater compassion and a deeper connection to my family and friends. I learned almost immediately who cared the most for me and who and what I really cared about and what really mattered. It has guided me on a path of insight and learning upon which I might not otherwise have set foot.

All of us, particularly young people, take our health for granted—until the day we don't have it. All young people feel that they are immortal—and some of us never lose that feeling.

That old adage rang through my ears: "When you have your health, you have everything." Suddenly, health takes on paramount importance in your life. This change in your health or your loved one's health opens up a new door and a new way of thinking that makes you appreciate every day that you live.

Before my diagnosis, I was an active young woman living a fairly healthy lifestyle. I did not drink or smoke. I got plenty of exercise. I ate a fairly healthy diet. However, the wake-up call of my diagnosis was a message that I could not ignore: Something had to change. I had to own MS, learn every possible thing about it, and trudge forward to get a grip on a disease with which I was unfamiliar. I would not allow that big dark cloud to take my life and independence away. I had two choices: I could continue living the life I had lived before my diagnosis, with the likely consequence that my condition would continue to deteriorate, or I could start over and create the life I wanted. I chose to listen to what my body was telling me. I had to embrace change, even though I thought I was already living a healthy life.

HEALTH IS YOUR CHOICE

No matter what your age, health is not a matter of chance—it is about choice, something to be achieved one step at a time and one day at a time, whether it's choosing the right physician to aid in your recovery or researching the many recovery options available to you. Changing your physical health, your mental health, and changing the people in your life requires hard work and lots of soul-searching. The good news is that all of us— young or old, healthy or ill, rich or poor—already possess the resources we need to get started. Nothing is standing in your way. The things you have to lose are the self-defeating habits of diseased thinking and preprogrammed responses that keep you from exercising your creative problem-solving skills. If you continually feel sorry for yourself and wallow in self-pity, it is a fact that your health will deteriorate so much faster than that of a person with a positive outlook. Instead, you can develop the life tools and strategies to build a solid foundation upon which you will create the life you want.

At that time in my life, I heard a quotation from Henry Ford that really changed my thinking: "Whether you think you can or you think you can't, you are probably right."

No health condition and no illness is insurmountable. Recovery begins by believing that you can overcome illness and live a productive and fulfilling life, no matter how devastating the diagnosis. I am a living example. Magic Johnson is another. So are Charles Schwab, Stephen Hawking, Teri Garr, Lance Armstrong, Andrea Bocelli, Michael J. Fox, and Muhammad Ali. The list is long enough to fill several telephone books. They are people of all ages and races from all walks of life. The one thing these notable people have in common is that they have not allowed their illnesses to dictate their personal successes or failures, and they have conquered impossible odds. The capacity for creating the life you want resides within you, and you must search deep in your soul to wake it up.

ENVISION THE LIFE YOU WANT

The mental leap I encourage you to take rests in your conscious understanding of who you are as a person and in taking total and unconditional responsibility for every aspect of your life, including your disease. Everything you do and think must be intentional: from the attitudes you hold concerning your condition to the physicians you select, the treatment plan you undertake, and the healing diet and exercise plan that will assist in your recovery. Especially important are your decisions about how you handle your personal life and your relationships. The sooner you can take responsibility for the choices you make and the healing attitudes you embrace, the sooner you can create the healthy life you want.

Do everything you can to remove yourself from unhealthy environmental conditions and emotionally toxic people, and do everything you can to work closely with your physician or physicians to aid in your recovery. This is common sense. However, the more challenging task is to take total responsibility for a medical condition that you didn't ask for, don't want, and sometimes can't control. There is no foolproof, absolute means to *will* your disease into submission. Changes take place on a cellular level beyond our reach. It may be difficult for you even to understand what is taking place inside you, let alone learn how to listen to what your body is telling you.

YOU ARE NOT YOUR DISEASE

Begin by understanding that you are not your disease. The cancer in your liver or the scars on your spinal column may, indeed, be a fact of your life. However, no one chooses cancer or Parkinson's any more than they choose their parents. I have MS, but it does not define who I am. Much of life is totally outside of our control. In the same way that not many of us are born with the talent to compose music or to add great sums of numbers in our heads, few of us are born with infallible immune response systems. Exposure to viruses and bacteria can be as random as earthquakes and tidal waves. They do not always target particular individuals.

The roots of the particular illness with which you have been diagnosed could be genetically hotwired into your DNA, or be a product of environmental factors totally beyond your control, or be a physiological condition related to trauma experienced in early childhood. There are many things we can do to prevent our health from deteriorating, such as not smoking, not drinking, not taking drugs, and not driving recklessly. However, despite all our efforts to live a safe and healthy life, sometimes disease strikes without explanation. There was nothing I could have done to prevent multiple sclerosis from attacking my body. Although I was already living a healthy lifestyle, I still needed to make more healthy choices—physically and mentally—to help myself fight this disease, and not allow myself to live around negative people who caused intolerable stress in my life.

Tempted as you may be to look back on past events and think that they should or could have gone another way, there is no point in such speculation. Blame and guilt are meaningless, an endless cycle of negative potentials leading you to identify yourself with your disease or condition. The positive is what you must embrace and keep in sight. You have been diagnosed with a life-altering or life-threatening disease, and whatever got you there is now in the past. From the moment of your diagnosis you must power forward in a positive, proactive way to do everything humanly possible to enjoy every day on this precious earth.

The most obvious choices you are likely to have made include the type of work you do, the food you eat, the exercises in which you engage, and who your friends and personal relationships are. Less obvious choices require deeper consideration. Many people with a chronic illness or debilitating disease chose to ignore small aches or pains, inklings or suspicions that something in the body was not right. Listen to your body.

Many people can watch a television show about good nutrition and then go out to eat twelve doughnuts. "I know it's bad for me," they may say, "but I'll eat it anyway." The smaller and seemingly inconsequential things people ignore, and the excuses they give, add up. If you are not mindful of the decisions you make, the recovery process can become a confusing nightmare of "what ifs" and "what might bes." The tasks I outline in this book—from facing your fears to choosing the right physician to dealing with the health care establishment—are methodical and goal oriented. They are directed specifically at expanding awareness of the options available to you and at enabling you to make the decisions that will prolong the quality of your life.

THINK POSITIVE

Surround yourself with positive people. If you are bombarded by friends, family, and doctors who all bring you down, eliminate them from your life. People who are surrounded by negativity tend to drown or to have tougher challenges trying to swim to the top. Your condition is difficult enough without having to feel that everybody around you is already planning your funeral. If people around you continually make you feel stressed out, you must separate yourself from them, because stress is a big reason for bad health and relapses. I learned the hard way that my marriage was impossibly stressful and definitely the roadblock to my ever getting better. Every book I read after my MS diagnosis said it over and over. I felt it slapping me in the face on every page I read—that with MS, stress will cripple you, kill you. If I had not listened and jumped out of my false comfort zone, I would not be functioning today.

I had to make one of the most important decisions of my life at that point. I had to get a divorce. I knew that if I did not, I would be confined to my bed and not be able to function as a real mother for my sons. If I was not there, who would be? I didn't feel as if I could count on their father. This thought destroyed me, while at the same time it empowered me to be realistic about the state of my marriage and to get divorced. I have never for one minute looked back and regretted this decision. I am living a full, healthy life now, and have been fortunate enough to marry an incredible man and to have been a full-time healthy mother to my three sons—something my doctors had not predicted for me. In addition, I recently gave birth to healthy and beautiful twin girls.

I do not encourage divorce, and I hope that every marriage can be a happy and supportive one. However, many illnesses rear their ugly heads when people are at the boiling point of bad relationships with their significant others. Eliminating that painful relationship frees you to have less stress and your body can begin the healing process. When you are ill, it's extremely hard to face the idea that your relationship is killing you, but it just might be.

Your focus will determine your attitudes, create your lifestyle, and ultimately determine the results. Energy flows where you focus your attention. Adopting a negative attitude—attaching blame to yourself, or thinking of yourself in terms of your disease—is a certain way of missing that important "turn in the road."

Taking total responsibility for your condition means that you must take control of the decisions about every aspect of your life from this point forward. You cannot crawl under a rock, hide your disease, and hope that by some chance or stroke of luck it will just disappear.

All people have the capacity to change their thinking—to change how they communicate, the mental pictures they hold of themselves, and, most important, their behavior. They can change how they choose to exercise their many health care options. This is what I mean about taking total responsibility for yourself. Everything you think, say, and do, from this point forward, needs to be deliberate.

Identifying the changes that need to be made and making the modifications are your responsibilities. Physicians and health care providers can help in the decision-making process. Very often you will get conflicting advice. However, the decisions themselves are yours, and only you can determine how effective those changes will be. Know going into the process that you already have the inner resources you need to make these decisions and to bring about change. Thanks to the catalyst of your illness, you have the motivation. This is the turn in the road you have to take.

FIND YOUR POSITIVE INNER CHILD

I am not a scientist, physician, or therapist, but I have learned through personal experience those things that promote the healing that you will want to bring into your life. Read over the statements below, and ask yourself, on a mostly true or mostly false basis, if these things pertain to your life:

- I am a generally positive person.
- I wake up in the morning with a sense of energy and expectation about beginning my day.
- I am happy about most of the decisions I have made during my life.
- I feel safe.
- I see the world as a happy place.
- I am making a positive contribution to this world.
- I feel lucky.
- I share decisions about my health with my physician.
- I am excited thinking about the future.
- I am a forgiving person.
- I see the strengths and good traits in my co-workers, friends, and significant other.

- I have plenty of energy.
- I am grateful for the help of friends and family.
- I am happy with myself.
- I eat nutritious foods.
- I am on my way to good health.

The above list contains just some of the many positives that can enhance our daily lives. If you have scored "mostly true" on at least ten of these statements, it is an indication that you are thinking in the right direction and are on the road to recovery. If none of these is true for you, you need to take a serious inventory of your life and see which things you can change. Choosing to change will, at the very least, empower you to embrace living with your disease in a positive and uplifting way. You may possibly outlive a very negative prognosis.

THE BEST WAY for each person to begin is by drawing up a new life plan. Who do you want to be? Where do you want to go? How are you going to get there? You may find it strange to be told to devise a new life plan when you feel as though you are at the end of your rope and are hanging on to your life, but this unusual proposal is actually the "lucky" opportunity you have been given. If there ever is a time in your life when you can conceive of a life plan with absolute dedication to honesty and to the profound insights that come from being faced with a life-altering diagnosis, this is it. The goal, simply put, is to achieve the greatest possible fulfillment and pleasure from your life.

EXAMINE THE STRANDS
OF YOUR ROPE

The journey you have taken has put you in the position where you really can examine the end of the rope to which you are holding on. Study the individual strands for what they are, and consider how well they have served you. Perhaps you will find that some individual strands of that rope are not as strong as they should be or that the rope needs replacing altogether. Perhaps you will find that the strands of your life's rope have been woven in such a way that they really will hold up under further stress. I know that some strands of my rope were not strong enough for me. Some completely snapped and let me down. This can happen to you, too. The rope, of course, is your body, and the individual strands are the many psychological and biological factors that strengthen or weaken it.

It is not enough just to imagine a new life plan, you must write it down on paper—keep a personal diary—describing exactly the life you envision yourself living. Make a list of the things that you would want if you could experience your life along new and different lines. Try to consider what you are doing as a preliminary step to the moment when you will push the reset button, as you would on a computer, and the program will start all over again. It may be more helpful for you to think of yourself as an artist about to begin painting on a new canvas, or a gardener planting seeds and bulbs in freshly overturned earth.

WHAT ARE YOU DOING
THE REST OF YOUR LIFE?

Start conceiving your new life plan. Now. Steal a few minutes to get started while you're waiting to see your physician, take notes on the back sleeve of an X-ray or MRI. No one is going to grade it. No one is going to compare it to someone else's life plan. This is yours and yours alone: a statement of what your life ought to be, could be, and will be. If it helps you to focus, write down your life plan as you would compose a letter to an intimate friend whom you have not seen for many years. Or write to a child who you hope someday might read and value the intimate letter you create.

Perfect health, unlimited financial resources, and loving relationships are naturally on or near the top of most people's life-plan lists. However, I want you to begin by identifying what actually is the most important: your purpose in life. Do not dwell on your disease. Just write down, as simply as you can, that which is most meaningful to you. Your purpose could include sharing your life's journey with a loved one, changing careers, running your own company, running a marathon, inventing a cure for disease, sky diving, or mastering the Internet. Perhaps you dream of a journey to the great sacred places of the world, or simply a closeness with nature.

I started taking karate lessons for the purpose of exercise and keeping my muscle memory intact after my MS diagnosis. I ended up loving how it made my body feel strong and took away my numbness and tingling. After five years of steady karate study with my friend Lynn Palmer, I earned my black belt.

You are ahead of the game if you know your purpose and have established your goals. If not, you must ask yourself what it is that gets you fired up. It certainly doesn't have to be your career. Your purpose may be found in caring for your children or in a hobby. It's the "why" behind everything else—that which makes recovery worthy of the effort.

JOSEPH CAMPBELL:
"FOLLOW YOUR BLISS"

Joseph Campbell, the great educator, author, and mythologist, advised his students seeking their purpose to "follow your bliss." He didn't tell them to follow their talents and skills, their social expectations, their egos, or even their happiness. Happiness wasn't good enough; he told them to look for bliss—those moments of ecstasy that transcend how much money a person has or where he or she feels the most needed.

Ask yourself, "What has prevented me from living out my passion?" The feedback you have previously received about the choices you've made will go a long way to helping you judge what has worked and what hasn't. The job or career you have chosen may bring you financial rewards, but it may have led you away from the life purpose that makes living truly worthwhile. On the other hand, your work may have become so stressful that you truly don't receive the psychological or spiritual benefits that drew you to it in the first place.

The same questions must be applied to other aspects of your life. The exercise regimen you have put yourself on may keep off a few pounds, but it may be no fun or may even be damaging to your knees and joints. Taking a brisk walk may accomplish the same health benefits without the trauma. The foods you have eaten may have tasted good, but may not have provided you with the nutrition that strengthens your immune system, that enhances your complexion, and that generates the energy you would like to have in your life.

Even if you cannot identify an ultimate purpose for which you wish to live your life, you can, at the very least, identify activities that nourish and strengthen your sense of self. Reading an uplifting book, hiking, entertaining, or spiritual contemplation are all good things to consider. You might decide to take a class at a local college, apply for a part-time job, or help a person less fortunate than you. Do not waste your time complaining—to yourself or to those around you. Instead, take action. You will create the life you want to live, one step at a time. As you build a house from the ground up, you build your life one brick at a time, but you must begin with a strong foundation, which starts with educating and empowering yourself.

EMBRACE CHANGE STEP-BY-STEP

Give yourself goals to accomplish with dates and times when you're going to do them. In later chapters we will focus on the specific steps you will take to jump-start your recovery process—such as choosing the right physician and making the medical care system work for you. Each task will be goal oriented and have a specific target date.

Taking on one giant task—a quantum leap, as Einstein would put it—is not the way to approach change. Divide and conquer your goal by setting up a step-by-step series of tasks. Each task must be manageable. I do not mean a routine or burdensome chore, but a manageable, incremental improvement that directly relates to your plan. Those tiny steps will add up to the quantum change. Nearly everything can be broken down into small tasks that can be accomplished one at a time. Day by day, little steps, small choices, and new habits combine to reshape you as a healthier person. Take that first step. As the joke goes, a person who does not try fails 100 percent of the time. Our great poet Carl Sandburg expressed this thought quite eloquently: "Nothing happens unless first the dream."

YOU ARE NEVER TOO OLD, TOO YOUNG, OR TOO BUSY

If your life purpose is to teach and you don't have a degree or credential, this could be one of the first things to include on your new life-plan list. Do not allow negative thoughts about your condition to stand in your way. There are always creative solutions. Instead of lying in bed with the TV remote control, read, search out the thing you have always wanted to do but never made time to do. You are never too young, too old, or too busy to chase your dreams.

START RIGHT NOW

One simple step toward taking responsibility for your life is to give yourself the Very Necessary Medical Identification Card that you will find on page 249 of this book. You need to fill in this card with your medical information so that it will be available at all times. This is vital information to be provided in emergency situations and very useful for health care providers in both emergency and nonemergency situations. Please fill it out, laminate it, and keep it in your wallet or purse. This is a good way to start taking charge right now.

∞

IF YOUR LIFE PATH involves growing spiritually, the same concepts apply. Get in touch with your inner self, or talk to religious leaders in your community. Find out about the power of prayer. From the first day I was diagnosed with MS, I have always said a prayer every night before I go to bed. I always start off by thanking God for everything good that is in my life and what has happened that day. Next, I pray for the things that aren't working and ask for guidance to make them better. My positives are much longer than my negatives. This prayer centers me and forces me to be realistic about my life and truly appreciate all that is positive. Perhaps you want to learn to meditate or to go on a spiritual retreat. Now is your chance.

If your plan is to learn to cook, do not allow something such as a wheelchair to interfere. Do your research. There are many kitchen alterations available for people with physical limitations. Take a cooking class and buy cookbooks.

If your purpose is connected to your family, you may begin simply by writing letters, scheduling quality time, doing genealogical research, or putting the family scrapbooks in order. If you have not already begun to tap in to the power of the Internet, you may be surprised by the extensive resources—the ease with which you can contact distant family members, trace lineage, and outline family trees.

CELEBRATE PROGRESS

Once you have made your life plan and have begun the journey, stop periodically to consider the progress you made at each step. Make a big deal and truly notice everything that works well in your life. People tend to magnify all the negatives when they have a life-altering disease. You cannot afford to ignore all of the positives and wonderful aspects of life around you. Celebrate each piece of progress, no matter how small. Check off the mile markers as you accomplish each task. Congratulate yourself, pat yourself on the back, and take time to relish the pleasure of those accomplishments. Doing so will enhance your ability to judge your progress and enjoy the change. Are the treatments you have undertaken enhancing your life? Are the decisions you have made changing your outlook? Are your relationships growing stronger? Are you, in fact, moving forward toward your ultimate goal? These are the questions you must ask.

If your plan is not working, alter it. Change the configuration or rethink the options available to you. Sometimes you will feel unhappy about how something is going but not know why. Take a closer look—you might find that some activity or goal is taking you away from another goal, such as quality time with friends and family. It is unlikely that every change will work perfectly. Continue to tweak your plan for change until you get it right.

Play detective. There are many twists, turns, and midcourse corrections. The idea is to create a world of possibilities. It's like starting a garden: you will plant more seeds than you expect to sprout, and nurture the ones that do. Feedback is what you want and action is what will take you there.

A determined woman named Diana McGowin wanted to write a book. The fact that she had Alzheimer's did not stop her—in fact, that was precisely why she wanted to write. Her challenges, naturally, were many, but she did it nevertheless. Today, proceeds from *Living in the Labyrinth: A Personal Journey Through the Maze of Alzheimer's* go toward medical research. Laura Hillenbrand, the woman who wrote the popular book *Seabiscuit*, which became a film, has Epstein-Barr virus (also known as chronic fatigue syndrome), and could not write more than a paragraph or two in a single day. Magic Johnson, who is HIV positive, has accomplished nearly as much off the basketball court as he did when he was playing. When Magic was diagnosed, we were all shocked and worried about how much longer the legendary basketball hero could live. Today, he is healthy, productive in business, and gives back so much to others.

This is a new life plan. It is yours, however unreasonable it may seem to someone else. If you are not working toward a new life, or at least a reconfigured life, then you really are bound by predetermined parameters. The turn in your road needs a goal, a series of landmarks to reach toward. Many people never seriously consider all of their life options, merely because they assume that those options do not exist. You do not have to feel limited by anything. Do not make this assumption. Find your dream. Do your research. Consider the telephone book of notable people with illnesses (see page 19) your inspiration. Lean on me and the life I have found. Let the healing begin.

Step One Summary

1. Create health by making good choices.
2. Live the life you want through deliberate choices.
3. Remove unhealthy environmental conditions—including people—from your life.
4. Distinguish yourself from your disease; make the distinction clear in your mind.
5. Embrace positive influences.
6. Follow your bliss.
7. Develop and reach goals: write down a life goal; then, a life plan; then, a series of tasks to reach that goal.
8. Give yourself deadlines and, as you achieve each one, celebrate.
9. Take action now.

STEP TWO

Fear Less

"THIS CAN'T BE HAPPENING TO ME. . . ." I have heard this refrain so often that I can guess what people are about to say by the bewildered expressions on their faces. It is exactly how I felt. Everyone I know with a serious illness has felt this way. My disease is MS. Other members of my family have suffered from diabetes, heart disease, Alzheimer's, and cancer. My friends have had all of the others, including kidney failure, brain tumors, and lupus. No matter which devastating disease strikes, the steps for dealing with it apply to everyone, and one of the first steps is to conquer your fears.

Denial, rage, anger, depression, terror, anxiety, and an overpowering feeling of helplessness are natural emotions to feel after receiving a diagnosis of a life-threatening or life-altering illness. When you add the sense of unfairness and the apparent senselessness of being struck down by a disease, the newly diagnosed find themselves totally overwhelmed and totally devastated. Quite naturally, you are in a state of fear, and the fears are many: the anxiety of not knowing what is going to happen; the uncertainty of not knowing whom or what to believe; the panic of feeling helpless in the face of seemingly insurmountable odds; the frightening prospect of facing your own mortality; the terror of trying to fathom how this will affect your family and loved ones; and the fear of wondering if you will still be loved or be hopelessly abandoned.

As frightening as these fears are, the more serious problem is actually your fear itself and the way it can immobilize you. The fear you experience in contemplating a diagnosis—or even in trying to summon the courage to seek a diagnosis—can be as damaging or more damaging than your disease. A delay in obtaining a diagnosis or in discussing the illness with a physician, and living in a state of denial, may in effect contribute to the very results you fear the most.

"Early diagnosis" is not a cliché: this can be a true matter of life or death. For many debilitating diseases the condition will, during these delays, progress from an early stage, where it can be treated, to a more advanced stage, where it becomes life-threatening and not as treatable. It is only through facing your fears that you will find a new strength and calm. You will discover that the reality of your condition is far less frightening than living with the sense of helplessness and hopelessness that comes with allowing fear to dictate how you live.

The intense flood of negative emotions that many people experience may also drive a wedge between them and the caregivers they need to count on the most. Turning your anger—a result of fear—on your physician or other bearer of bad news interferes with the exchange of vital information that may save or prolong your life. The tendency to withdraw into ourselves is a natural consequence of fearing the unknown environment in which we find ourselves.

From acne to cancer, the body responds directly to what we think. This is not some alternative health theory, but clinical fact. Many leading physicians will go as far as to say that how we respond to stress is the single most determining factor in overall physical health and in the chances of a patient's recovering from a serious or life-threatening illness.

THE PHYSIOLOGY OF FEAR

Fear operates on a profound physiological level. The chemical reaction that fear sets off in the body influences how it responds to infections and, for example, the hormones that determine such life-sustaining conditions as blood sugar levels. Feelings of anger, anxiety, tension, and depression have been shown to produce high blood pressure and to increase hormone levels, lower the immune response, constrict arteries, and contribute to a host of other conditions that give rise to and perpetuate illness and disease. In contrast, feelings of joy and gratitude as well as laughter have been proven to lower blood pressure, reduce hormone levels, and boost the immune response.

In the course of work with my foundation, I typically get three or four calls each week from people newly diagnosed with MS or some other life-threatening illness. From their tone of voice, I can usually tell how well these people will do in fighting their disease. People who have great attitudes, even those with the most horrendous symptoms, do remarkably well—especially if they lead very busy lives. When I talk to people who have negative attitudes—the ones who are all doom and gloom—I emphasize the importance of attitude. Right from the start I counsel them to face their fears and not to say, "Poor me. Poor me. My life is over." I encourage them to realize that this is the only life they will ever have. They have to live it to the fullest every single day and cherish every moment that they feel well. I tell them that they must take the steps to educate themselves back to good health.

Everyone, of course, experiences fear. That fear is hot-wired into our systems. The resulting adrenaline and cortisol pumped into our bloodstream sharpen our motor and cognitive skills in life-threatening situations that require quick and strong responses—to save ourselves from a car careening toward us out of control, for instance. Fear provides the burst of energy we need when it matters most.

The release of these stress-related chemicals triggers two responses from our bodies. The release of adrenaline is called the "acute alarm" response, which gives us strength to stand and fight the problem at hand. The release of cortisol is called the "chronic vigilance" response, which provides endurance to flee the problem or problems creating the stress. Taken together, these two responses make up the body's fight-or-flight response. They are the body's way of protecting us from harm, but when we overreact to stress we expend much more energy than the problem requires.

Any person faced with a chronic illness will naturally feel a mixture of sadness, anxiety, and depression. This is completely normal. Your challenge is to face that fear and overcome it. Don't let it eat you up. Do not allow your disease to become the label of you as a person.

During times of stress, adrenaline can stimulate the release of glucose—which in turn can negatively affect our pancreas, our weight, and our energy, or lead to hypoglycemia, in which blood sugar levels are too low. Stress is also the biggest drain on our vitamin and mineral levels. It weakens the immune system and can contribute to life-threatening illnesses—perhaps the one you are dealing with right now. In fact, stress can kill.

It is clear from clinical studies that corrosive effects of long-term stress wreak havoc with our mental and physical health. This can be true even without a life-threatening illness thrown into the mix.

The potential damage of stress is always present in our lives. A daily injection of fear-based imagery into our conscious and unconscious minds can have a devastating effect on our health and sense of well-being. One of my main goals in writing this book is to help you to educate yourself thoroughly about your disease. This knowledge will give you a more positive personal approach and enable you to confront the intimate fears connected with life-threatening illness. I wish such information had existed for me fourteen years ago, when I was first diagnosed.

The emotions that I experienced when I was diagnosed with MS ran the gamut—from denial that I actually had a disease, to intense rage that the universe had somehow selected me as its latest victim. "Why me?" I cried out inside. As many people experience, the relentless emotional pain of feeling helpless and distraught was coupled with daily physical numbness and lack of feeling. One fed off the other, threatening to engulf my life. I felt as though the foundations on which I had always stood had suddenly crumbled. I lost all sense of time and proportion. Things that seemed meaningless before my diagnosis took on greater importance; things that were once important seemed inconsequential. Rage and anger, the fear-based emotions that have the most detrimental effects on the body's immune system, flared out of control. Sometimes I became foggy, not hearing correctly what the doctor was telling me about what was really wrong with me.

THE MANY FORMS OF FEAR

Each person, of course, will experience fear differently, and the manifestations of fear may appear in different forms. Fear of dying is naturally foremost for all of us, followed by fear of pain and fear of being incapacitated. There could be fear of financial failure, fear of the loss of quality of life, or anxiety over family adjustments that will inevitably have to be made. Marital problems and potential divorce can emerge as the result of a life-threatening disease. The triggering mechanism for fear can be the loss of the ability to drive, to enjoy sexual intimacy, or to run a marathon. The chronically ill may fear not only the loss of motor skills but a future that they are no longer able to predict. Your familiar routine will no longer exist.

Decisions become more difficult to make because the odds have changed. You may ask yourself if the investment in energy and time it takes to accomplish a task or to take a particular direction is worth the struggle. This can lead to depression and a host of other, equally insidious emotional conditions.

This is where denial comes into the picture. Denying that you have a disease and refusing to consult a physician or undergo treatment becomes a way to avoid facing life's more important challenges and questions. Only through the process of facing these fears and exploring the "whats" and "whys" of your condition can you learn the effective coping skills you need.

These skills will enable you to lift yourself out of what appear to be overwhelming situations. Most important, letting go of fear permits you to access your creativity and the empowering skills that will be necessary for your recovery. Fear can be so smothering that it becomes impossible for you to tailor creatively a treatment plan that is right for you as an individual.

Your creative will is the single most important tool in reclaiming your life. And that will is not impaired by illness. Your

own creative impulses about how to approach a particular challenge, and how you are going to meet that challenge, will determine your ability to formulate and stick to a treatment
program. Physicians, medical practitioners, and friends can
help, but you are the only one who can determine what is the
right course for you to take. In this and every other step outlined in this book, please remember that you are the most important player in the healing process. *You* have to make the
decisions. Only *you* are in a position to decide your future. To
give in to your fears is the same as handing your life over to the
people and institutions that know the least about you.

For me, and for most others diagnosed with a serious illness,
the basic cause of the outpouring of fear is unavoidable. I had
the disease. Simply stated, I could not step back in time and do
things differently. I decided, however, that I was not going
to play the victim and take things sitting down, or, as my
physician suggested, lying down (TV remote in hand). The
drama taking place in my house was not going to be television
tragedy. I was going to face my fears—as all of us must who are
seriously ill.

The program for facing your fears is task oriented. It involves
taking control over your life, one step at a time. First, you must
identify and define each of the fears you are grappling with. Do
not just dwell on them. Divide and conquer them by writing
them down. Make lists and keep a journal. Address the fears
one by one as unfamiliar objects, as if they were the contents of
an old home that needs remodeling to be livable.

Stockbrokers might think of their fears as plummeting financial indicators. Artists may think of them as a collection of
ugly canvases. Choose the imagery that is most meaningful for
you. It does not matter what metaphors you choose; the important part is to find a mechanism, such as list-making, that will
help you name and confront your fears.

Once you have made your list, step back and examine your notes and ask yourself how much better your life would be if the drab furniture, downward financial indicators, or ugly canvases were replaced with more positive images. Try to imagine how you would spend your life if the fears of death, pain, family turmoil, or financial strain were not factors in your life.

KNOWLEDGE IS POWER

The best antidote for fear is knowledge, and knowledge, as has often been said, is power. Knowledge of who you are, where you want to go, and how you can become educated about your illness or condition will be the most powerful tool you have at your disposal.

Fear of a life-threatening disease can be turned into a call for positive action. Take a closer look at exactly what it is you have to fear. Is it death? Perhaps, but none of us is going to live forever. Life is a terminal illness—nobody gets out alive. We may not have control over how long we live, but the quality of life we choose to live is everything. Want to start taking positive action right now? Turn to page 249 and fill out the Very Necessary Medical Identification Card. Laminate it and put it in your purse or your wallet. You will have taken an important step to protect your health in many circumstances, but particularly in medical emergencies. Of course, there is much more to do.

It is time to reflect positively on all the things that you want to do in your life and to take action. Perhaps you have always wanted to learn a foreign language, go mountain climbing, take a trip around the world, get to know family members better, or spend time with a childhood friend. If you think of it positively, your diagnosis may actually not be the curse it first seems to be: it could serve as a wake-up call to stop putting off the things you have always dreamed of doing. It may be a signal to rearrange

your priorities. Some of the most important contributions made
by artists, musicians, and scientists the world over have been
produced amid debilitating, chronic, or terminal illness.

The challenges presented by a life-threatening illness often
invite positive changes when you reach out toward unrealized
dreams. Relationships that were once unfocused and self-
destructive are given up or become rock solid. A sense of
peace and tranquillity can replace a life of chaos and turmoil.
Remind yourself that you are lucky to be alive still and be grateful for the opportunity you have been given to realize your
dreams.

REACH OUT AND SHARE
WITH YOUR LOVED ONES

The possibility of hurting my children and loved ones was
for me a great anxiety. Many people are so consumed by this
particular fear that it prevents them from informing their loved
ones of their illness in a timely manner, or from telling them at
all. However, this is a time when families can become much
closer. The realization of how precious and important the bond
is between you and your children and loved ones becomes
vivid.

Here again, to banish your fears, make a list, or write in your
journal. Be specific. Avoid generalities. Write an explicit and
detailed account of exactly how you feel your illness or condition may harm the people you are most concerned about. As you
do so, you may find that the impact you think your condition
will have on loved ones has less to do with them than it does
with your own pride and ego. For me and for many others on the
long journey back to recovery, the act of sharing the experience
with those who love us provides opportunities for growth—not
just ours, but theirs—far beyond what we might imagine.

The most meaningful approach is always the team approach. Rather than make your illness a barrier to your relations with others, consider it a bridge, an opportunity to reach out to loved ones and for them to reach out to you. The opportunity for their personal growth can be as great as yours.

Some people are very secretive and go to great lengths to hide the truth. This can also add to your stress. I just decided to take the plunge and tell everyone right away. There was a barrage of phone calls and I-feel-so-sorry-for-yous, and many people just looked at me with great pity. Some friends were afraid to hug or kiss me or even shake my hand, for fear that my MS might be contagious. Where I live, news travels really fast. Everyone heard, gossiped, and reacted—and then it was accepted and I could begin my healing without that extra element of having to hide my deep dark secret.

Telling everyone gave me a great sense of relief, but many people have a legitimate reason to try to hide their illness. They fear going public about their diagnosis because there is a very real chance that it could affect their livelihood. They might not get hired, or they might lose their jobs or not get promotions. Even nurses in hospitals have had to hide their illnesses for fear of losing their jobs. Although this applies to many occupations, it is especially true in Hollywood—I know several actors who are hiding their illnesses because they fear being labeled as unreliable. It is common for actors cast in TV pilots to sign a six-year contract, ensuring their commitment to the show if it gets picked up and becomes a success. Many actors and actresses can't afford to let people know about their illnesses because to do so would genuinely hurt their chances of be hired. This is so unfair and greatly adds to their stress.

RENEW THE BONDS
OF LOVE AND DEVOTION

The effect that your condition may have on your spouse or lover is another serious concern. You may fear that your mate will abandon you. He or she may not be psychologically prepared or capable of handling the role of caregiver, or may simply desire to be with someone healthier. However, a crisis such as this is more often an opportunity for partners to reveal the depths of their dedication and love.

In addressing this issue you must ask yourself if the lover or mate you have chosen is actually the right life choice. Overwhelmingly, you will discover that the support and the depths of love revealed will surprise you. However, you may find, as I did, that regardless of your health, you may not wish to share your life with someone who does not recognize a mutual commitment. Your wake-up-call diagnosis may actually be a blessing, because no one deserves second best. Unconditional love is the most potent weapon you or anyone else has to fight disease. A true loved one will share your pain equally with you. Your mate is a part of you, and what hurts you truly hurts him or her as much if not more. Your loved one will be your partner in every way and your absolute best support system.

COMMUNICATION AND SHARING
WITH LOVED ONES

Communication is a vital part of dealing with such issues. Half of this responsibility is yours. The people who love and care about you the most are those who need to be kept informed. Moreover, keeping secret your fear of a medical condition is a losing proposition. Those who know and love you will notice the subtlest changes in your demeanor and behavior. The likelihood is great that your family will misinterpret what is taking place. Secret medical appointments may be misconstrued as avoidance or lead to the suspicion that you are hiding something much worse than your diagnosis.

Diseases affect families and close friends, not just individuals. Remember that your family and friends are suffering with you. You need to share information and make them part of your healing process. Realize that you are not a hero when you refuse to be honest; in fact, you are selfish if you do not share your struggle. Your loved ones are the very people you will need and want to count on for support. They need to be advised about how you are feeling. And if you have been diagnosed, they need to know what to expect.

Children are especially sensitive when something is wrong. Their world completely revolves around them, and they feel responsible for everything that happens. Without information, they may blame themselves, thinking that something they said or did has put Mommy in a bad mood, or that Daddy doesn't love us anymore. They need to participate, and to become familiar with the strange and perhaps scary changes in your life: new routines and responsibilities, changed moods, and even medical equipment you may be using.

When I was diagnosed, I was terrified that I might say the wrong things to my children. I consulted a child psychologist, who told me that the right approach needed to be tailored to the age of the children. My boys were then 6, 8, and 10 years old. He told me that it was important to be completely honest with them but not technical in my description of MS and its manifestations. He wisely observed that there was no point in dwelling on the worse-case scenarios for either me or my children. I truly didn't want to scare them.

Remember, you are your children's primary teacher. They will look to you for direction. If you do not wince at the sight of a needle or feel queasy from hospital odors, chances are that they will not. You need to approach the subject as you would if you were giving them a lesson—and to think of it exactly that way. It is an opportunity for them to understand how their bodies function, and how to handle experiences when they themselves are ill, injured, or hospitalized. Make sure also to inform their teachers so that they, too, can help your children come to terms with what you have just told them.

This is above all a lesson in compassion—you are teaching your children how to treat people who have an illness or are disabled. Do not make your children or spouse feel guilty about your disease. They did not cause it and they do not deserve the guilt. If you are dishonest with them, even just once, they may not trust you ever again, and very possibly might feel that you are much sicker than you are.

ALLOW YOUR FAMILY TO HELP AND SUPPORT YOU

Fear of being helpless and losing your independence may be directly related to the anxiety you are feeling about your family and loved ones. You must define exactly what it is that you are frightened of losing and how you think this will impact you and those who love you. I dreaded the thought that my children might one day have to push me around in a wheelchair. It is natural to feel that this is a burden you would not wish upon anyone, least of all the people you most care about.

What I did not realize was how much strength I gained from their love and support. From the moment of my diagnosis, my mother and father moved into action and came to my side.

My children were especially wonderful, particularly when I allowed them to express their love and support for me. Now that they are older, they have become more involved with my multiple sclerosis fund-raising event and have soldiered on in the fight to erase MS. Every year they introduce me on stage and give a very heartfelt talk about me and MS. Your feelings of love for your children do not change. No matter how old they are, let them express what is in their hearts. Relationships are often strengthened in unforeseen ways. Learning to care for, and to be cared for, is often a healing process for all.

Know that whatever your disease may be, it becomes a family disease. Everybody now has it and suffers for you. You are not alone in your diagnosis, and therefore you cannot be selfish enough to make decisions only thinking of your best interest.

In some cases, people who have been diagnosed with a chronic illness dwell on the "why me?" It is reasonable to be angry about the unfairness of the situation, but not reasonable to think that you can't do anything about it. There wasn't a big list of diseases one day and you chose one. You do not choose to have a disease. The disease chooses you. There is no point in feeling guilt for having contracted a disease. This is a self-punishing mechanism that erodes your sense of self-worth and competence. If you can, forget about fairness or the deserving and the undeserving. Put it behind you. Life just does not operate on those terms, no matter how much or how often we wish it would. The important thing is to accept it and move forward.

The mind-set you should strive for is simple: There is no failure, only feedback. Life is a game of trial and error. People learn from their experiences. It is important to think of your diagnosis as the wake-up call that it is. Your test results become, in effect, a work sheet you can use to examine your options and reconfigure your life path.

Like many of our other psychological issues, the difficulty you may experience in dealing with the "why me?" feelings of victimization is conditioned by the preconceptions you or

those around you have about your disease. This is especially
true for smokers who have contracted lung cancer, or diabetics
who have been unable to adhere to regimented dietary restrictions. The resulting "blame game" accounts for some of the
worst psychological abuses by the chronically ill and by their
health practitioners.

COUNTER THE "BLAME GAME"

To counter the "Blame Game," you might begin by listing the
things that people have advised you to do, and then carefully
consider them one at a time. Often "learn to adjust" may be
code for "resign yourself to poor health" or "settle for less than a
desirable existence." These messages have no benefit and will
be impediments to a proactive attitude. You need to be forth-
right in telling others that no matter how sympathetic they
feel, they are not giving positive support when they tell you to
stop fighting. Also, you may find that statements such as "just
stop feeling sorry for yourself" completely miss the point of
what you are experiencing. There is truth in how and what you
feel.

People are naturally inclined to assume that when good
things happen to them it is because they made good choices or
did the right thing. A "good" child earns a "just reward." Conversely, when misfortune strikes, people tend to think that it is
a result of "bad" behavior. The truth, however, is that none of
us is in total control of what happens to us and it is a mistake to
act as though we are. You can no more control the many challenges life is going to throw at you than you can control the circumstances of your birth. Accept the fact that all people,
doctors and patients alike, have problems. A person who has
not had challenges has not really lived or experienced the true
depth of the human condition.

REMEMBER: THERE IS NO FAILURE, ONLY FEEDBACK

A more subtle kind of fear you may be experiencing involves your friends and their genuine outpouring of affection. I have known sick people who withdrew from their friends and loved ones at the very moment they most needed their help. The conscious or unconscious fear you may be experiencing is helplessness—you don't know how to respond to the attention and affection they are showering on you. You may receive stacks of get-well cards that you cannot begin to answer. Your message machine may be overloaded with calls from people whom you feel obliged to call back, but you do not have the energy to talk to them.

In evaluating these issues, you must try to identify exactly what circumstances bring on your feeling of helplessness. Then deal with them individually. Each challenge will require your own creative solution. People want to help, which is why they are sending the cards and making the calls in the first place. You should allow them to express themselves while you take a few practical steps to keep yourself from being overwhelmed. Delegate responsibilities. Consider putting a friend with a good telephone voice in charge of taking all incoming calls, and have your phone service forward your incoming calls to him or her. A simple act like this produces many benefits. You increase your peace of mind, knowing that someone is responding to efforts to reach you, and at the same time you gain the space you need to step back and take care of yourself.

A year before giving birth to my twin daughters, I lost a baby when I was six months pregnant. I went for a regularly scheduled checkup and my doctor told me that there was no heartbeat. My baby had died inside of me, for no known reason. I had to go through two days of painful labor and delivery. I was also overwhelmed with grief—I simply couldn't face telling this story over and over again, so my close friend Lynn Palmer called and told all my friends. She asked them not to call me or come to the house for a while because I needed privacy to mourn this devastating loss. Everybody respected that and gave me time to deal with my feelings. We all do things in our own way, and at that point I was far too emotional to keep telling my story.

Lynn's help and support meant so much to me then, but it was also a way for her to show her love and concern for me. Actions like this give a friend or family member who really wants to help a chance to do so. At this point in your life, you should take advantage of all the positive love and support you can get, but beware of friends and family who are negative. Distance yourself from those who persist in a negative attitude about your condition. Other people's unrealistic fears can be very toxic to you and can harm your prognosis. Surround yourself with people who have a healthy outlook on life.

TERI GARR, MS. SPOKESPERSON

Actress Teri Garr is a close friend of mine. She has an Academy Award nomination, but for a long time she had trouble acknowledging that she suffered from multiple sclerosis. Today she is a brave and articulate spokesperson for raising awareness about MS, but for many years she exhausted herself worrying about what people would think of her condition. She feared that admitting that she had MS would hurt her ability to get hired. Fear of being labeled with a disease is another common self-limiting condition that prevents people from moving forward.

Before I met Teri at a fund-raising event in Aspen, I had heard through the grapevine that she might have MS. Some people in the entertainment business mistakenly thought her outward changes were signs of a much worse disease. There was one interview in particular on *The Tonight Show* with Jay Leno. She stumbled when making her entrance, which raised eyebrows, but the cause was her MS.

The Aspen event presented me with an opportunity to talk with her about multiple sclerosis and the experiences I'd had. Although she opened up to me a bit about the strange physical symptoms she was having, she did not at that time completely believe she had MS. My heart went out to her. Teri had a young daughter and her marriage was crumbling. In the years to come, she would have difficulty walking. I recommended some unbelievable MS specialists to her, and kept telling her the importance of exercise, which she heeded on and off but never truly committed herself to. Despite being such an amazing actress, she had trouble getting film roles, and she was constantly fatigued.

This was the very thing she feared the most—not getting the right starring film roles—and it came true, not just despite her efforts to hide her disease but in some measure because of them. Teri's fears prevented her from seeking help in a timely way. More than ten years elapsed before she really decided to face MS and start fighting the disease. Although I and others recognized her symptoms right away and gave her advice, she didn't truly accept the diagnosis of what was wrong. She kept telling me that she wasn't sure. "Maybe it's MS and maybe it's something else," she would say.

Today, Teri Garr responds as I do when friends express pity. "Don't feel sorry for me," she tells them with her famous radiant smile. "With your help, something can and will happen to turn my condition around." More colorfully, she has adopted the slogan "MFMS." She has truly become an inspiration and an advocate for people with MS, and she speaks all over the country about living with the disease. With her light and humorous approach she has been responsible for helping thousands of people accept their MS and become educated about the many positive steps they can take. She has enriched her career and now her personal health in the most meaningful way.

It is natural to want to avoid having a disease label attached to you. People are more likely to pity you. "Oh my God, Nancy, I'm so sorry," friends would say to me. I don't fault their good intentions or the sincerity of their feelings; however, the mere display of pity shuts doors that need to be opened. It is natural for friends and loved ones, and even physicians, to define us by our disease: "She's the MS girl." They do so because they have been shaped by the climate of fear, the frightening images of illness, and cultural prejudice. You do not have to let them do that to you. You are *not* your disease. Gently remind them that you welcome positive support, but do not need negative sympathy. They will get it.

Shock, fear, and denial are natural reactions following a diagnosis. The challenge is to move past those reactions to acceptance and treatment. By acceptance I do not mean "adjustment" or "giving up." I mean accept that you have the disease and begin to move forward, actively exploring your options to reconstruct yourself—spirit, mind, and body—in new and improved ways.

Your life will never be as it was before. In some ways, it may actually be better: more cohesive, focused, appreciative, and perhaps more loving. Look for the best-case scenario, and reach for it one step at a time. Your response to chronic illness must be task oriented and team driven. You must learn to say, "Today I will walk as many steps as I can," or, "Today I will read and learn more about my illness." Each step must be celebrated as a victory. The attitude I established for myself is one of gratitude for the opportunity to move forward. I ask for nothing less from myself and those around me. Meet the negatives with a positive. Let joy take the place of fear.

Step Two Summary

1. Verify and then accept your diagnosis; the prognosis is up to you.
2. In your journal, make as long a list as possible of your specific fears.
3. In that same journal, keep notes on how you faced and conquered each fear.
4. Consider your positive response to each fear and how you can use that response to benefit further. Do not tolerate negativity within your close circle of friends and family.
5. Use your creative will to see new ways to embrace and enhance your life that will dispel your fears.
6. Reach out and share experiences with your loved ones, and fight the anxiety about evolving relationships.
7. Teach those around you how to support and improve the life you are building with simple tasks, such as answering your telephone.
8. Do not allow anyone to define you by your disease; you are the same person they have always known and loved—not an object of pity.
9. Move forward every day; seek new ways to build strength and confidence in your journey toward health.

STEP THREE

Never Take No for an Answer

EVERY MORNING I begin a ritual that I have practiced for the past fourteen years. I sit up slowly so that I do not become dizzy. I carefully bring one leg at a time over the side of the bed, placing one bare foot on the ground to make sure I can feel the floor solidly under me. Then I put down my other foot.

The best days are when I am able to stand up on my own with complete feeling in both legs. There is nothing better than the sensation of my own two feet grounded on terra firma with every part of my body awake and working as it should be. "Thank you, God, for another day of independence!" I say to myself. I celebrate such days by standing quietly for a few extra moments before I begin my day. I remind myself that I am blessed, and I feel appreciative of the fact that, at least for this day, I have the strength and independence to hold myself tall. Knowing this makes me smile all over and leads me to appreciate all that comes next: the sun shining through my bedroom window or the children whose photographs sit on my dresser. It is an exercise in letting go of fear by appreciating what I have. It is also about setting goals and finding something that motivates me to move forward when the odds are stacked against me— about never taking no for an answer.

Never taking no for an answer is the most positive affirmation you can make to yourself. It is a declaration that you are not going to give up, give in, or give way, despite how unfair and unreasonable life seems. I am saying, in essence, that whatever happens to me, I can cope with it. I have to take charge, and remain in charge, even when I am not feeling well. I have set goals according to what I can accomplish and given myself a reward, even if it is only taking time to look at pictures of my children and realizing just for that moment how truly lucky I am that I can simply stand.

Instead of dwelling on the pain, I consider the many things in life that bring me joy. I accept my condition, but I say no to the limitations and restrictions by affirming: "I am not able to do some things just now, but I am going to build from the ground up and do what I can." One of my favorite sayings comes from Norman Cousins, who was diagnosed with ankylosing spondylitis and given just a few weeks to live. He survived—and thrived—for more than twenty years thereafter, and lived by the motto, "Accept the diagnosis, but do not accept the verdict that comes with it." I say my own version of these words of wisdom every morning: "I have MS, but MS doesn't have me." I have a life that I fight for every day.

In the same way as overcoming your fears can jump-start the healing process, there is dramatic clinical evidence of the impact that a positive attitude has on survival rates. Among patients with such debilitating conditions as metastasized cancers, those who expressed greater hope at the time of their diagnosis survived longer. The patients attributed their success to a broad range of causes, but only one factor was common to all cases—a more positive attitude.

Cousins described the preliminary findings of a national survey of oncologists while he was at UCLA Medical School: More than 90 percent of the physicians said they attached the highest value in fighting cancer to the patient's attitudes of hope and optimism. The same findings were true of AIDS patients and others with debilitating diseases. The patients who maintain a positive attitude, or who take charge of their lives, do best. Their "will to live" means that they really want to live and are willing to do whatever they can to squeeze more quality out of it.

FOCUS ON WHAT YOU *CAN* DO

Total control over your life, of course, is not possible. Regardless of your condition, there are circumstances and events imposed on all of us that we cannot predict, did not cause, do not want, but are altogether unavoidable. It is difficult to know, in advance, how our bodies are going to react to a particular medication or treatment, when our illness may flare out of control or go into remission, or how our loved ones are go-ing to react. In the case of MS, symptoms develop unpredictably. No two patients are alike, nor does the disease follow the same course in each person. You must be prepared by keeping yourself informed about what you can expect, listening to what your body is telling you. Keep abreast of all the latest medical developments, and make decisions that are right for you.

Just as you worked to overcome your fears, it is essential to maintain a fighting spirit throughout your hardships. People who have a fighting spirit are not frightened of dying because they know what they are up against. When and if that time comes, they are at peace with it. They have accepted, genuinely and unconditionally, that they are not their disease, and hence, they are not ashamed when they do not look or feel their best. Equally important, they take total responsibility for their health by taking charge of their options. They do not allow others to make the decisions for them because they view themselves as active participants with a fighting spirit in combating their disease or illness. They are not victims, but active participants with their medical support team in their fight for improvements, remission or cure.

WHAT *CAN* YOU DO TO FIGHT BACK?

"Can't" is another way of saying "no," and you are not accepting that attitude. Sometimes, in your darkest hours, you may have difficulty in thinking about what you *can* do to fight your disease. Here are some suggestions:

1. You can read, think, and absorb information. An extraordinary part of your health can be found in the mind/body connection. Engage your brain; do your research; focus on positive options that you can begin today.

2. You can become an active partner in the search for your health. Ask your doctor how you can help him or her. Bring ideas to your appointments. Ask questions. Take notes.

3. You can communicate with others who share your health problem or who have overcome it. These may include friends, co-workers; or people you meet in the pharmacy or in the doctor's office, and you can learn from all of them.

4. You can experiment with options you may never have tried before to connect with your body and thereby become better able to hear what it is trying to tell you. Meditation, prayer, yoga, relaxation therapies, stretching exercises, and diet variations are just a few of the possibilities to explore.

5. You can carefully record your thoughts, sensations, and medications in both a medical and a personal journal that can be unexpectedly useful to you and your doctor. If you take the time to write them down, you may be surprised by the details you remember. It is also very therapeutic to put it all on paper.

∽

MEDICAL SCIENCE may not yet have found a cure for your illness or disease, but there are always options available to you. Sometimes your options may not be pleasant or easy, or they may come with a heavy price. However, know that there are always options to be exercised—regardless of your condition, and regardless of what a doctor may tell you. It is entirely up to you whether or not you choose a particular treatment, medication, or therapy. For example, you may choose the comfort of your bedroom and your loved ones for caregivers rather than a lengthy stay in the hospital.

Investigations on your part may reveal that the pills you have been prescribed or have been led to believe are "treatment" for your illness are meant only to mask symptoms, not to treat the disease itself. Advice and counsel from people who have coped with or overcome the disease you are living with may be more meaningful and ultimately more helpful to you in developing a treatment plan than the agenda your physician or caregiver has in mind.

TAKE CHARGE OF
YOUR HEALTH CARE

Take charge over what is happening to you. Know going into it that you already possess everything you need to assume the undisputed leadership role in your health care. It is a matter of turning your potential into a reality, and doing it one day and one step at a time. No one can manipulate your emotions and behavior in making you choose a particular path unless you permit them, which truly well-intentioned loved ones may try to do.

The first, and perhaps most important, step is to recognize your own boundaries, and the many ways and means that physicians and the health care system use to assert control over you. Understanding the language that medical practitioners employ is the starting point. Terms such as *incurable*, *inoperable*, *untreatable*, *life expectancy*, and *hopeless* are, by their very definitions, words that limit a patient's expectations and, by extension, his or her options. You have the right to walk out the office door of any doctor who uses this kind of negative terminology and gives you no hope. I know many people who have done just that.

The physicians and medical practitioners who use such language are sometimes officious and intimidating. In many cases, the mere presence of a physician and the language that he or she uses makes patients feel powerless, passive, and withdrawn, and therefore less likely to ask the questions that may save their lives or to speak up for themselves. *No* does not have to mean *no* in every case.

Take a cue from the younger generation—look at how children react to "no." Generally they are very curious and driven to turn no into yes—especially if it's something that matters greatly to them. For children, the word "no" is often little more than a temporary impediment, a stumbling block. They often relentlessly revisit the issue (much to their parents' frustration), introducing new options and hypothetical situations; more often than not they eventually turn no into maybe and finally into yes. In that same way, be creative, and, yes, persistent with your doctors—there's always something you can do, *always*. In essence, revert back to the strength of your child-hood.

Intimidation is a special problem during hospital stays. Upon admittance, you are asked to surrender the trappings of your individual identity—your clothes, valuables, purse, and wallet. Rather than permit you to wear your own clothes, they give you a flimsy hospital gown that barely covers your rear end, and an ID bracelet, which makes you a number in the hospital system. You may be sharing a room with a total stranger. The attitude with which you confront such depersonalizing circumstances may determine your survival. The solution to maintaining a positive attitude may simply be to bring your favorite robe, pillow, or blanket into the hospital with you, or to decorate your room with family photographs. You may wish to bring some music that makes you feel relaxed and a portable CD player or other device to play it on. Never set foot in a hospital without a health care advocate—a friend, a family member, or, if necessary, a hired professional—by your side. Bring all of your personal medical records, X-rays, and blood results with you as well.

SEEK HEALTH AND RECOVERY

Dwelling on the worst-case scenario is perhaps the fastest route to becoming one. People can and do recover from "incurable" diseases and "fatal" illnesses. Sadly, the people most likely to fulfill a prognosis of a six-month life expectancy are those who have been told—and believe—that six months is all they have.

I am aware of several instances in which people I knew were diagnosed with an incurable form of cancer, given a short life expectancy, and died right on schedule—precisely when their physicians told them they would. The shocking truth discovered afterward was that they didn't actually have the particular illness their physicians had diagnosed. The power of your mind is absolute.

Don't ever give in to a time limit for your life. Any doctor who tries to predict one for you should be cut off at the pass. My father proved to me the wisdom of this approach—over and over again. He recently passed away, but throughout his life he survived a number of serious illnesses, many of which we were told would be fatal.

I remember when he was diagnosed with double pneumonia and was hospitalized at UCLA. He was quite ill—doctors told us that there was an 85 percent chance that he would not survive. The rest of us were depressed, but true to form he walked out of there four days later—against doctors' orders—and went straight to work.

He proved his doctors wrong many times over a fifteen-year period because he always had the strongest will to live—no matter what anybody told him. Unfortunately, a combination of symptoms took his life two days before my twin daughters were born, but I learned such a valuable lesson from him. He loved everything and every minute that his life had to offer. He never complained about feeling ill, because he didn't want to burden anyone around him. His zest for life and his tough fighting spirit probably added an extra ten years to his life. He lived every single day to its fullest like nobody else I have ever witnessed.

My father beat the odds time and time again. His doctors often told us that he was a medical miracle, but to me it was never a surprise. With so many health issues stacked against him, it was his strong and indomitable will to live that gave him so many more precious years on this earth and with his friends and family.

Do not let your doctor play God for you. You have a right, an obligation, to say no. Expect that it will be difficult to exercise this right—especially when you are feeling sick, worried, and stripped of the many things that make you feel like a competent adult. Nevertheless, you must take charge and vigilantly maintain control over your person and your environment. Always ask what the treatment options are available to you. If you have a problem or are not receiving the care you have every right to expect, be prepared to take a step up the ladder of the medical bureaucracy until you get the health care to which you are entitled.

Have no illusions. The medical establishment deliberately makes any review procedure or protest time-consuming and difficult. They want patients to give up. Your job is to be relentless. Continue calling and writing until you are satisfied. The first notice of benefits denied will come from your health care insurance company in the form of an "explanation of benefits," or EOB. More often than not, the "explanation" is incomprehensible, so your first line of defense will be a discussion with the customer-service department. Sometimes, this may result in a clearer explanation of why payment was denied. Whether it does or not, you will be required to submit an appeal in writing. This appeal will be most effective if you have a discussion with your doctor's office to discover alternative ways to present the bill for service. Be sure that your letter is accompanied by a copy of the EOB in question—this contains all of the pertinent information and code numbers for the insurer.

Our federal government has no mechanism to deal with insurance company denials. Happily, forty-two states and the District of Columbia have review boards. Usually, these boards include physicians who may be more familiar with treatments for various conditions than are the insurance company employees who have issued the denial. If you are not able to find satisfaction with the review board, you have no other alternative than to take the matter to court. Often, simply the prospect of a trial will stimulate an out-of-court settlement.

The reason why physicians are likely to describe conditions such as my father's in such pessimistic terms may actually have nothing to do with a personal diagnosis. In fact, it may have little to do with medicine at all and much more to do with the law—specifically with limiting the exposure of your health care provider or your doctor's insurer in case of a malpractice suit. Advising a patient of the extreme downside—the worst possible outcome, the most extreme symptoms, and the least likelihood for recovery—lessens the grounds for a malpractice suit. Physicians in many cases are mandated to paint a gloomy picture, as they have been trained to do in medical school. These schools, like the health care system at large, were once part of a healing tradition dedicated to maintaining health, but have now evolved into being part of an industry that emphasizes illness. Because of the need to protect themselves legally, the entire system is now rigged in such a way that risk takers—physicians and caregivers searching for solutions outside the norm—are challenged at every turn.

THE DANGER OF MEDICAL SPECIALIZATION

The rise of specialties, such as cardiology, neurology, dermatology, orthopedics, and psychiatry, has further removed physicians from considering the overall health and mental well-being of their patients. Attention has been diverted from the intrinsic interrelatedness of all parts of the human body and the complex dynamism of a person's own immune system. Illness is multidimensional, and the treatment of illness must be, too. Proper health must be recognized as a balance of many inputs, including physical and environmental factors, emotional and psychological states, nutritional, and exercise.

In the medical system as it exists in our country today, a specialist in one field doesn't necessarily know or care to know what another is doing. Knowledge, diagnostic tools, and treatment can be fragmented. Many diseases, such as cancer, are labeled or identified by particular organs, although a particular cancer is likely to be the result of an imbalance in another part of the body. The emphasis on specialties, and the money that these subcategories generate, creates a one-sided system in which the true underlying cause for a disease or an illness is often overlooked. Also lost is the concept of helping a patient to reconfigure his or her life—whether it is changing diet, detoxing the system, or just getting enough rest and relaxation. Problems in these areas can sometimes be identified as the elements that allowed the illness to occur in the first place. All too often, the symptoms, not the cause, are what is being treated. If at all possible, find a quarterback doctor who assimilates all the doctors and medicines into one.

A physician cannot, of course, single-handedly rewrite hospital mandates that have been determined by a battery of attorneys. It is up to you to become informed and to speak up— to ask questions when things happen that you do not understand and to insist that your feelings and opinions be considered. Despite the many sensitive and optimistic doctors who practice compassion, a sad truth is that there are many others who deliver a dreaded diagnosis with no sensitivity to the patient on the receiving end. A patient can easily become intimidated, and can forget that his or her life hangs in the balance.

Patients receiving a life-threatening or life-altering diagnosis are poorly prepared—emotionally and psychologically—to hear such pronouncements, or to judge for themselves the efficacy of a recommended treatment. A patient will already be at a profound disadvantage because he or she is debilitated and is overwhelmed by the symptoms that brought them to the physician's office in the first place. At the same time the patient's life is unraveling, the physician doing the diagnosis is cool, calm, and collected. These physicians are in their own element. They have years of experience and often do not mind telling you so.

You can find yourself accepting the worst-case scenario when you should be declaring, "No, this is not going to be me," or, "No, I am not going to accept life in a wheelchair." At times of crisis and heightened emotional upheaval, people can barely comprehend what is being said to them at all. They leave the physician's office thinking, Six months . . . Or thinking as I did, No cure, no hope, no life. Depression and withdrawal, the net results of these experiences, have no benefits for survival. Nor does sitting at home with the TV remote control all alone wallowing in self-pity.

BETTER WAYS TO DIAGNOSE

The doctor/patient relationship does not have to be this way. In the best of all worlds, a physician would replace negative medical jargon with language that uplifts and builds: *renewal, rejuvenation, wellness,* and *hope.* The kind of scenario I would like to see is one in which a knowledgeable physician has thought out, in advance, how best to present the results of tests—and there are many doctors who will do this. Rather than have a nurse or aide on hand to run interference, or to guide the patient out of the office, this doctor might have someone in a nearby waiting room to talk to you, someone who has been on the receiving end of a similar diagnosis and has defied the odds and safely returned to tell the story. At the very least, your physician should lay out a plan for wellness directed toward em-

powering you to take control over your disease. I'm not talking
about sugarcoating a diagnosis, but rather directing a patient's
attention to the many positive options that are available to him
or her. When doctors truly don't have any answers, they should
be honest and tell you so, and if necessary refer you to someone
else.

HOW TO REWRITE YOUR DIAGNOSIS

Imagine a scene in which your doctor has taken the time to
consider a presentation of medical news to you that will
help and support you in the months and years to come. Create
the dialogue in your mind or on paper according to these concepts:

1. Clear, conclusive diagnostic tests show that you have a
serious health problem; however, there is plenty of hope. We—
doctor and patient—begin today on a journey back to health,
and we will explore every avenue of cure and control until we
find the one that works for you.

2. You can help by educating yourself about your health
problem. Here is a list of books and Web sites that will give you
useful information.

3. There are many choices, many options for you to consider in your journey of rejuvenation. Here are a few for you to
look at, and I hope you will find others that we can consider together.

4. I will offer opinions and give you the benefit of my experience and knowledge; however, the final decisions about your
treatment are up to you. I need all of the energy and commitment you can give to help you fight for your life.

5. I will spend all of the time you need right now to answer
your immediate questions. Then, there is a former patient wait-

ing in my office whom I would like you to meet. Three years ago, she was given the same diagnosis I just gave you. Today, she lives a happy, normal life and her health problem is under control. I think you can learn from her experience.

6. Listen to your body; it will be the best guide for both of us in this journey.

Unfortunately, rarely is a diagnosis delivered in the positive manner I have described above. Nevertheless, there still exist many incredible and thoughtful doctors who do, many of whom I have been fortunate enough to see. That said, it's up to you to do your homework and seek them out.

∞

PATIENTS ARE GIVEN MISINFORMATION or incomplete information on a daily basis at almost every stage of the journey—by physicians, by caregivers, and even by loved ones who subtly try to manipulate the patient into following a particular agenda or by doing what they feel is best. The inherent problem here is that your decision about what is best for you will not always neatly coincide with that of your physician, his or her medical practice, or the hospital where you have been admitted. The close and sometimes intimate relationships between products and their salespeople often create a conflict of interest for the doctor. A pharmaceutical salesman is not the best judge of a product any more than an auto-parts salesman is. Stop and consider, if you will, how long it took before seat belts were mandatory on automobiles.

Because of insurance requirements, most doctors are given a time budget that mandates how long they can spend per visit with each patient. In most cases it is not long enough to talk about all the possibilities, give a diagnosis, go over test results, discuss new medications, *and* spend time dealing with the emotional component of your disease. This is truly not their fault, so it is very important to make every minute of your doctor visit productive. Go in with your well-thought-out list and don't leave until your questions are answered.

DO NOT BE MANIPULATED

Manipulation can be as subtle as your spouse or significant other telling you that "the doctor knows best," or as extreme as a physician planting unreasonable doubts in your mind that may result in your undergoing surgery. It happens all the time. Your only defense in this and similar circumstances is to keep yourself informed at every step of the way. Knowledge is power! The more educated you make yourself, through reading, second opinions, and discussions with others who have had the same disease, the better you can make your own decisions. Learn everything you can about a surgical procedure before you ever go under anesthesia. Make sure that you have the best surgeon, one who has performed your operation many times before. There is no need for you to be the guinea pig.

Topping the list of your bill of rights is something that no physician, caregiver, or significant other should ever violate: your right to judge your own behavior, thoughts, and feelings, and to take responsibility for them. In other words, you have the right to be in charge. Just because you are ill and fighting a disease does not mean that you are any less capable of determining your future or cannot creatively find solutions that are right for you. It is your future, not theirs.

Just because a treatment has been successful for one person does not mean it will work for you. Always ask how many times your doctor has performed the procedure you are considering—and what the results were for the patients. You must ask: How many people were helped by the procedure? How many had adverse side effects? How many have died?

The same right extends to all phases of your treatment and interactions you have with physicians and medical practitioners. I have provided a copy of the Patients' Bill of Rights later in this chapter. No one is permitted to touch you, give you an injection, operate on you, force you to take medication, or even change a bandage without your permission. You cannot be held in a hospital against your will. No one can force you to accept a treatment you don't want, even if a nurse or physician says that it will save your life. The choices are yours to make.

The important part is that you must make your wishes known. Open your mouth and ask lots of questions. Be politely assertive and you will gain much attention and respect. You must ask the questions you need to ask and do not stop asking them—politely—until every question has been answered to your satisfaction. Before you have a surgery or any other major procedure performed, look on the charts, look at your X-rays, and check your ID bracelet. Is the staff preparing to do the same surgery that you discussed with your doctor? Is he or she focused on the correct part of the body? This may sound silly, but there are many documented stories about the wrong limb being amputated or the wrong breast being removed because of mistakes or a fatal dose of the wrong drug being given because of inattention. Unless you speak up, physicians and medical practitioners will assume that your permission is implied by your presence in their office or in a hospital. Never take anything for granted.

I have a very close friend who recently underwent spinal surgery. As he began to feel the first relaxing effects of the anesthesia on the morning of the surgery, it occurred to him to look at his chart. To his horror, he read instructions to operate on the T3 and T4 vertebrae. Having been following carefully discussions of his spinal problems, he knew that the operation was supposed to be on T1 and T2! Because of a discussion the two of us had just had, he was informed and in charge, and he saved himself from a mistake that might have left him paralyzed. No one else was there to do it for him. You have to do it for yourself, too: You must be in charge of your own medical care and never become complacent.

PATIENTS' BILL OF RIGHTS

Although it was the subject of great debate in 2004, the United States Congress, under considerable pressure from corporate health providers and insurers, did not adopt the Patients' Bill of Rights. You should request a specific statement of your rights from your health care provider, doctor, or hospital in your state. However, most physicians and hospitals endorse the following principles:

1. **Respect and nondiscrimination:** The patient has the right to receive considerate and respectful medical treatment without discrimination as to race, color, religion, gender, national origin, disability, sexual orientation, or ability to pay.

2. **Participation in treatment decisions:** The patient has the right to be informed, in accurate and easily understood language, of all information about diagnosis, treatment, procedures, and medications for their plan of care. This includes the right to make decisions about all treatment options and the right to refuse treatments. This also includes information about the identity of doctors, nurses, and others involved in the patient's health care.

3. **Confidentiality and privacy:** The patient has the right to every consideration of privacy. This includes the right to talk in confidence with your health care providers and to have your health care information protected. You also have the right to review and copy your medical records from both your physician

and your hospital and to request that your physician change your record if it is not accurate, relevant, or complete.

4. **Advance directives:** The patient has the right to have a living will, health care proxy, or durable power of attorney for decisions concerning his or her health care. Physicians and hospitals must honor the terms of these directives to the extent allowed by state laws.

5. **Pain control:** The patient has the right to adequate pain control and the right to choice of pain-reducing drugs.

6. **Research:** The patient has the right to consent or to decline to participate in research studies or experimentation affecting health care. This right includes visitations by medical students in teaching hospitals.

7. **Visitors:** The patient has the right to authorize family and other adult visitors for hospital visits. In most cases, this includes the right to have an advocate by the patient's side at all times.

8. **Facilities:** The patient has the right to clean and healthful hospital facilities and personnel. You are entitled to a smoke-free room. This includes the right to complain without fear of reprisals and to anticipate a prompt response from the hospital. This usually includes the right to request transfer within the facility or transfer to another facility, if feasible within the restrictions of your health care insurance.

9. **Emergency care:** The patient has the right to prompt admission to emergency services, stabilization, and necessary treatment whenever and wherever needed, without prior authorization and without financial consideration.

∞

JUST AS YOU HAVE the right to say no to a procedure or medicine, you have the right to know the identity of all the doctors, nurses, and other practitioners involved in your care. It is not uncommon to find that you have agreed to have a specific physician treat you, but that he or she has assigned a student, resident, or other trainee to take that doctor's place. This may be unacceptable to you. As a patient, you are entitled to high quality hospital care delivered with skill, compassion, and respect.

In the case of surgery, one of the operating room doctors that not enough patients meet is the anesthesiologist. His or her job is to suppress your nervous system enough to keep you from feeling pain during the operation. He or she also must keep a close watch on your blood pressure, pulse, and breathing. In other words, while the surgeon is performing the procedure, the anesthesiologist is keeping you alive. You will want to talk to and feel confident in this person, who literally holds your life in his or her hands for the duration of the surgery. You should interview this person before you ever go to the hospital. If possible, make sure that you like your anesthesiologist and that he or she knows your allergies and any complications you've had with previous surgeries or with any painkillers. They also need to consult with you about your allergies and weight. If you weigh much less than a normal person, the prescribed amount of anesthesia will be overwhelming and could cause bad side effects. The same is true if you are overweight; you may need more anesthesia for the procedure.

You are also entitled to a clean and safe environment while being treated. The greatest mistake you can make is not speaking up when you are receiving substandard care. This can range from a nurse or physician not washing his or her hands before touching you, to your physician failing to explain the medical consequences of what he or she is doing.

NO NEED TO EXPLAIN

Another important right you have is to offer no explanation, reason, or excuse for justifying the decisions you have made. No explanation is necessary because the option you have chosen to exercise is your own to make, and you are willing to live by the consequences of that decision. Just remember that everything you do will be trial and error. It is the feedback that is important. Your feelings may at times be irrational, but logic is not the goal. It is a matter of respecting your feelings. Remember that you—not your physician—are in charge of your body.

The decision you make may simply be that you are not ready to move forward with a particular treatment or life choice. Adopting a wait-and-see attitude is not the same as doing nothing. Rather, it is "watchful waiting." When you are being pressed to make a decision on the spot, don't be afraid to ask for a little more time to think things through, do a little more research, or get another opinion. This may be the case in choosing to undergo chemotherapy, to be placed in a nursing home, or to make decisions regarding your financial resources. Some procedures have very negative "side effects" that are not always explained completely. Perhaps friends or loved ones are pressuring you to create a living trust, or to turn your assets and power of attorney over to them. You have the right to say that you are not ready, or that however "unwise" your decision might prove to be, it's still your decision to make.

You also have the right to withhold permission for expensive testing. Just because your health insurance provider will pick up the tab does not give them control. Their participation sometimes can mean that you are paying an emotional, physical, or psychological price much higher than the money.

The phrases *I don't know, I don't understand,* or *I don't care* may be the most powerful words you have to defend your position. However frustrated your physicians, caregivers, or loved ones might feel in your saying these things, they will eventually get the message and become less assertive or manipulative toward you. Rather than alienating the manipulator, opening lines of communication by expressing your feelings in this way is disarming. It may take time for your message to sink in, but when it does you may be surprised at the result. Many times, physicians who have resisted you the most become your partners in the recovery process. And the best way to strengthen this partnership is to extend and share it with others. The emotional experience of sharing supports your love of life, your will to survive, and the intimacy you will feel with all your caregivers, be they family and friends or medical specialists. Take the time to appreciate all the doctors, nurses, and other health care givers. They have a very tough job. Thank them; write letters to let them know how important they have been in your time of need. Many times the really good ones don't receive the accolades that they so richly deserve.

WRITE IT DOWN

Merely asserting yourself and adopting a positive attitude, however, is not enough. Listen to and write down what is being told to you, then go home and do your research. You have to know what you are talking about, and you have to learn to speak the language of the health care system. Learn the facts of your illness. If you are given a statistic, learn its source and how old it is. Find out if you are being given the whole, unadulterated truth or only the information that has been selected by your physician, perhaps to guide you toward a certain decision about your treatment. In considering your treatment options, keep in mind that it takes years, sometimes decades, before a new treatment or procedure becomes included in textbooks, and longer still before it is generally accepted by the mainstream medical community. This doesn't mean, however, that the treatment has not been tested or written about. Study the medical journals to find the latest research.

When I was diagnosed with multiple sclerosis fourteen years ago, there was no Internet where I could look up information about my disease. There was no known cause and no known cure for MS, and no clear protocol for how to live a healthy life with MS. Fortunately for me, my great friend Brenda Richie, who is now the Internet queen, went to the library and painstakingly copied hundreds of pages for me from selected books. It really helped me understand and get current with the latest research so that I could truly understand my illness, when so many doctors had told me there was no information available.

Many people will naturally feel overwhelmed at the prospect of reading and understanding medical journals. Here is where a health care advocate may be the solution—a good friend or family member who will help you to understand what's going on from a medical standpoint and join you in meetings with your physician. Your advocate doesn't need any special expertise regarding your condition, only the ability to ask the right questions and the willingness to comprehend and then translate medical jargon. He or she must have the time to listen to your physician and the patience to deal with the medical bureaucracy. You may discover, as I did, that the job is too big for any one person, and that you will need to recruit several people, each of whom will bring a different expertise to the table.

Just as you made an inventory of your fears, make a list of the questions that come to mind about your disease. This learning process may be the most important education in your lifetime. There is no such thing as a stupid question. You are in a new and perhaps unfamiliar environment, and it is naturally difficult to deal both with the rigors of treatment and with educating yourself at the same time. If you encounter a difficult article, make a photocopy of it or highlight the passages that don't make sense and ask your physician to explain them to you.

Here again, never take no for an answer. You are the consumer in the equation. It is your health that is at risk, not that of your physician. Do not allow your doctor to imply that he or she is doing you some kind of personal favor or to treat your request for information as if you were asking for a loan rather than for medical expertise. You are entitled to know exactly why your physician has prescribed a particular medication or treatment, what the side effects might be, and what alternative treatments or medications are available to you. Again, keep a paper trail of what you learn. Details that did not seem important at first may take on new significance later on. If you are successful in your treatment, you will want to know what those details were.

SEEK FORWARD MOMENTUM

As important as these and other resources will be for you, the most important is your body. Listen to what your body is telling you, not to what other people may say. No one knows you better than you do; no one knows what "feels" right to you and what does not. Remember that a medication or treatment that is right for one person will not necessarily be right for another. High doses of painkillers may do more damage than good. I personally hate taking painkillers after a surgery. They make me nauseated and give me terribly disturbing nightmares. I get off them as soon as possible. I'd rather have the pain, but each person has a unique pain threshold and a unique life situation. Factors such as quality of sleep, nutrition, muscle conditioning, and even body temperature play a role in how various pharmaceuticals may affect you. Only you will know when something is not right, because it does not feel right. You have more options than simply to put up with inadequate or ineffective treatment. Continuously, you must seek forward momentum.

It may at first be difficult to listen to your inner voice. I know it was for me. There was so much other noise that I couldn't hear myself think. I had to take myself to a separate place—both a physical *and* a mental place—before I heard anything at all.

Carry this over into your recovery process. You will have to say no to everything that diminishes your life, your options, or the vision of the person you see yourself becoming. Only by doing so can you say yes! to those things that enrich, enhance, and nurture.

Step Three Summary

1. Be positive; say Yes! to a better life.
2. Focus on what you *can* do.
3. Take charge of your life and especially your health care.
4. Knowledge is power: educate yourself about your health.
5. Do not be manipulated or intimidated.
6. Know the Patients' Bill of Rights.
7. Demand time to think, and ask questions if you don't understand.
8. Write everything down: keep meticulous files of all medical records and discussions.
9. Listen to your body: it will tell you everything you need to know to be healthy.

STEP FOUR

Find Your Dr. Right

∞

THE DAY AFTER MY EARTH-SHATTERING DIAGNOSIS, I went immediately to get a second opinion from a multiple sclerosis specialist at UCLA Medical Center. "Have you ever had any tingling or numbness that you can recall before this recent episode?" he asked.

"As a matter of fact I did have problems. . . ."

I explained that for the last seven years I had experienced a curious phenomenon: Whenever I leaned my head forward I felt numb from the waist down. As soon as I lifted my head, however, the numbness went away. The experience was so disconcerting that I had visited a neurologist seven years earlier. After several neurological tests he assured me that I had nothing to worry about. I never asked for a second opinion, even though I continued to experience these symptoms off and on for such a long time. I did not want to be perceived as a hypochondriac.

Instinctively, I knew that something must be seriously wrong, but again I ignored my intuition. That highly respected neurologist from one of our most prestigious hospitals had missed an important sign of MS: Lhermitte's syndrome. The electric tingle and numbness that characterizes this syndrome is often triggered by movements of the neck.

I paid a heavy price for not trusting my gut instincts and seeking a second opinion. It was a mistake I would never repeat. Now, I always consult more than one medical expert when something goes awry. In my search for my Dr. Rights, I am careful to choose physicians in a methodical way. I find recommendations through word of mouth. Most important, I have trained myself to ask the questions that really matter.

Unless you live in a big city, you may not have access to a wide range of physicians and specialists. And in many cases, HMOs and managed health care plans choose the medical team to work with you, or at the very least narrow the field of available options. This does not mean you cannot find your Dr. Right. You must educate yourself on what your choices are and you must take charge of the decision-making.

Dr. Right exists for you. He or she will be compassionate, kind, brilliant, and attentive to your needs and concerns, and will want to include you as a partner in your treatment. Physicians of this kind generally do not advertise their services or have toll-free telephone numbers, so it will be up to you to find them, no matter how much your HMO or the medical bureaucracy tries to interfere by playing gatekeeper and matchmaker. Finding the right doctor will require research, even hard work, but following a few simple guidelines may save you from making a costly and dangerous error.

HOW TO FIND DR. RIGHT QUICKLY

- Begin by looking at a teaching hospital or research clinic that specializes in your medical problem. The doctors will be well educated, focused on your medical issues, and knowledgeable about the most cutting-edge information.
- Educate yourself about your disease and prepare a list of questions for your prospective Dr. Rights.
- Be candid, assertive, and demanding in your interviews. Be clear about your expectations. You are hiring someone to help save your life.
- Find a Dr. Right who has a positive outlook, a person who takes the time to explain medical procedures in language you can understand. Be sure that he or she understands that this relationship is a partnership and that you will make the final decisions about your life.
- If you wish to explore alternative therapies, be certain that the doctor is open to those possibilities.
- Make sure that the doctor is open to second opinions and ask him or her for referrals. Self-confident doctors welcome a second opinion and are not threatened by it.
- Ask the doctor if he or she is aware of clinical trials that may be promising for your medical problems, and does he or she have access to such trials?
- Be clear about the level of communication you require. How quickly and by what method will your questions be answered? Is there an emergency telephone number answered by a live person that is available twenty-four hours a day? Will the doctor trust you with his or her home or cell phone number?
- Always ask nurses and hospital administrators who the best doctor in your field is, or whom they would go to if they had your illness.

- No matter how perfect the first doctor you interview may seem, interview at least two more doctors, time permitting. You need a framework of comparison to find Dr. Right. Check with friends and people you know in the medical community. This may be the most important decision of your life.

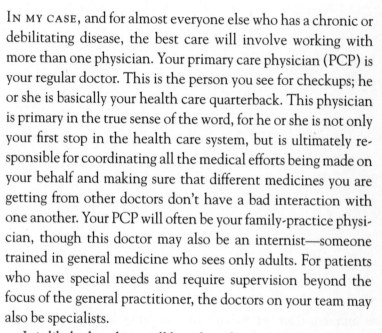

IN MY CASE, and for almost everyone else who has a chronic or debilitating disease, the best care will involve working with more than one physician. Your primary care physician (PCP) is your regular doctor. This is the person you see for checkups; he or she is basically your health care quarterback. This physician is primary in the true sense of the word, for he or she is not only your first stop in the health care system, but is ultimately responsible for coordinating all the medical efforts being made on your behalf and making sure that different medicines you are getting from other doctors don't have a bad interaction with one another. Your PCP will often be your family-practice physician, though this doctor may also be an internist—someone trained in general medicine who sees only adults. For patients who have special needs and require supervision beyond the focus of the general practitioner, the doctors on your team may also be specialists.

It is likely that there will be other physicians caring for you. If you have a stay in a hospital, an attending physician will be in charge of your care there. He or she may also be your PCP, depending on which hospital you are staying in and the problems for which you are being treated. More often than not, this physician will have had a history of working with you. If you have heart problems, your attending physician may be a cardiologist, or for cancer, an oncologist. A third type of physician who may see you is a hospitalist, one directly in charge of your care if you are admitted to an intensive care unit (ICU). Hospitalists work in teams or units and are present twenty-four hours a day in the ICU, so that nurses do not need to contact your attending physician or PCP and wait for a call back to take immediate action. Hospitalists rarely see patients once they have been discharged.

A TEAM OF SPECIALISTS AND SUBSPECIALISTS

Finally, your medical team will likely be made up of a host of other specialists and subspecialists. Each will bring his or her particular expertise in a variety of areas. Most common are radiologists—doctors who specialize in reading and interpreting diagnostic X-rays and other imaging techniques—and anesthesiologists, who administer medications or other agents that relieve or prevent pain, especially during surgery. For people who have chronic or debilitating diseases, many other specialists may be necessary: dermatologists, physicians concerned with disease and disorders of the skin; ophthalmologists, whose specialty is treatment of the eyes; neurologists, whose concern is the central nervous system; and immunologists, who study and treat disorders that involve the immune system. A subspecialist is different from a specialist in that he or she has completed training in a general medical specialty and then has taken further training in an even more specific area of that specialty. Cardiology, for example, is a subspecialty of internal medicine; pediatric surgery is a subspecialty of surgery. Understanding who these people are and what they do will be important in your ability to put together the right team for you.

HOW TO SELECT THE RIGHT PCP

The physician you will want to focus on at first is your PCP. The procedure for picking a PCP who is your Dr. Right is similar to the selection process for other doctors; however, your primary doctor has some special issues that need to be addressed. For example, you probably already have a primary physician, and you may be quite pleased with the care this doctor provides. Your relationship with him or her may go back years, even decades. This person may treat other members of your family. More often than not in today's insurance-driven system, your HMO may have chosen your PCP for you, or asked that you choose one from an approved list. No matter how you obtained your PCP, it is still important to check on this doctor's credentials and become familiar with how his or her medical practice operates. Although this could be uncomfortable, your life may depend on it.

Your PCP is the quarterback of your entire health care program. He or she usually will make referrals to the specialists who will be on your team. He or she will be able to gain inside information about those specialists and other medical personnel, knowledge that is often difficult for a layperson to acquire. There are many important reasons for having the utmost confidence in your PCP, even when you are consulting internists or other specialists on a regular basis. Your PCP will likely be the physician who knows you best and can put together all of your concerns in one logical package. And knowing you best—including your activities and your home environment—allows him or her to act as your advocate in questions or disputes you may need to clear up with your HMO, insurance company, or hospital personnel.

A SMALL TEST FOR YOUR PCP

A useful—and revealing—question for you to ask a prospective PCP might be: What information would he or she like to have included on your Very Necessary Medical Identification Card (see page 249). His or her answers might suggest the depth of thoughtfulness about emergency medical issues and might add to the value of your card. Whatever happens, you will learn something about how the doctor you are interviewing thinks.

THE FACT THAT YOUR PCP IS LICENSED and is legally entitled to practice medicine is not an indication or endorsement of his or her knowledge, skills, or experience. A physician is licensed to practice general medicine and may earn added recognition in a particular area, which is called board certification. This certification is conferred by your state board of medical examiners, after a doctor passes a state or national medical examination. Each state has its own procedures to license physicians and sets standards for all physicians in its jurisdiction.

KEEP IN MIND that you are not buying a new car or a kitchen appliance. This is your life you are enhancing with your frontline medical adviser. It will be up to you to find out how good a doctor's training has actually been, what former or current patients have to say about the doctor, and how his or her particular medical practice operates. Naturally, you will want to know how often the doctor attends medical conferences to be updated about the latest findings in a particular field of medicine, and if he or she has written any recently published articles. If a doctor does not take the time to learn of the latest new procedures and new drugs, you may be cheated of the best medical care for you, since things are constantly evolving.

ALWAYS ASK TRUSTED SOURCES

The first step in selecting your PCP should always be to ask trusted sources—family members, friends, colleagues or co-workers—for recommendations. However, you must remember that these opinions are based on your source's personal experiences, and not everyone you talk to will have an objective view. They may unknowingly be getting substandard care—or they may be in such fine health that they have never had reason to be especially demanding about the quality of their health care. You must judge for yourself—if a physician has a personable and reassuring manner, and can communicate comfortably with you, then that's a plus. That said, it is more important that he or she is skilled and well educated in the latest medical procedures. Sometimes, for example, you may find a surgeon who has a lousy bedside manner but a stellar reputation. If that doctor regularly performs a large number of the type of surgeries that you need and has a high rate of positive outcomes, he or she might still be Dr. Right for you—despite not being Dr. Congeniality.

Nurses, and to some extent hospital administrators, can be a great source of recommendations. They are medically knowledgeable and will likely be part of the larger network of nursing staff whose livelihood rests squarely on their working relationships with a variety of physicians and specialists. Nurses often know who is the best, whom they would go to, and whom to avoid. They generally have nothing to gain or lose by giving you an honest on-the-job opinion of what they have learned. A good way to open a dialogue with a nurse might be to ask which physician he or she would see if they were in your shoes, or, for that matter, which doctor they see now. You might also ask doctors you know to whom they send their family members.

The Dr. Rights you will be looking for are most often those described as "bright" or "caring" and who take a personal interest in their patients. They will be physicians who tend to call ahead before their patients visit a hospital, who closely monitor their patients while they are in the hospital, and who encourage the nursing staff to notify them, day or night, if something seems out of the ordinary.

Another important step in researching your PCP is to check whether any source has rated that physician's skills. Although a *Consumer Reports* for the medical profession does not yet exist, basic information on doctors in certain states is available for a small fee at www.docboard.com, a Web site run by a group of state medical-board examiners. Another source is a series of "Best Doctor" guides from Castle Connolly Medical, Ltd. This organization publishes *America's Top Doctors: The Best in American Medicine* as well as several regional guides. *Who's Who in Medicine and Healthcare* is also an informative guide. These books are available at many libraries and bookstores and through Amazon.com.

If you or someone you know is able to access the services of www.bestdoctors.com, you will find this a valuable resource. At the moment it is available only through employers or health care insurance providers. Founded in 1989 by Harvard Medical School–affiliated professors, this service rates doctors in all medical specialties based on independent evaluations by other doctors. Only thirty thousand doctors in the United States— less than 5 percent—qualify for inclusion, and they are reviewed on an annual basis.

In consulting these sources, however, care must be taken in

considering statistics and other information you may find in them. For example, just because a surgeon has low mortality statistics does not guarantee that he or she is one of the best surgeons. Shocking as it may seem, some senior surgeons have been known to place juniors in charge of high-risk operations and designate themselves as assistants on the surgical report for the purpose of evading responsibility if a patient dies. On the other hand, a very good physician may often take on high-risk patients, people turned away by other physicians, and hence will have a higher mortality rate.

Perhaps more important than what statistics may reveal is the history of where and when the physician attended medical school and served his or her residency, including any further advanced training and routine updating of knowledge through reading, watching tapes, or attending seminars. Often, this information is available directly from the physicians or their staffs. If you encounter any difficulty in obtaining this history, that may be reason enough to strike the physician from your list of prospective doctors. Some doctors may have begun without solid training, or may have dubious credentials; or their staffs may lack the standards of knowledge or cooperation you will want to receive. In either case, if you have doubts, you must trust your instincts. Whenever I fail to listen to that inner voice, I pay dearly.

HOSPITAL AND MEDICAL SCHOOL RATINGS

Once you identify the school or institution where the physician trained, your next step is to find out how highly that school or institution is rated. The *U.S. News & World Report* Web site, www.usnews.com, is one such place to consult regarding medical schools and training hospitals. Most libraries have at least one reference book that provides information about the pros and cons of each medical school or residency program. If a physician has published articles in medical journals, especially on subjects directly related to your condition, it is a bonus.

In most states, you can also check whether lawsuits or disciplinary actions have been filed against a physician. This data is often in the public domain. The risk-management departments of many hospitals list this information, as do state medical boards. However, just as the statistics you will find in physician-rating guides may be misleading, legal records can be difficult for a layperson to read and understand. A physician may be sued even if he or she did nothing wrong. Malpractice lawyers often name as many defendants as possible—regardless of the extent of their involvement in a case. A doctor you are considering may have been only marginally linked to a case that ended in a suit. Further, insurance companies may choose to settle a case even when no wrongdoing took place, simply to avoid a costly court battle. Another mitigating factor may be the degree of risk in the procedures that the doctor undertakes—a cardiovascular surgeon is likely to have been sued more often than an allergist. Age and experience are also factors—a doctor may have a clean record merely because he or she is relatively new to the profession. Any young doctor with many malpractice suits, however, is a red flag.

MEET OTHER DOCTORS IN YOUR PCP'S GROUP

Learning about the medical group your prospective PCP belongs to also gives important insights into options that may be available to you. A large, multispecialty group practice, for example, provides a patient with easy access to specialists and other medical personnel. Even if you do not intend to consult other physicians in the practice, find out who they are, what their medical backgrounds are, and evaluate how comfortable you feel with them. It is probable that one of them will be handling your case when your PCP is on vacation, involved in the care of another patient, not on call, or otherwise engaged. In all fairness, doctors deserve some private time, and after regular office hours only one doctor in a practice is normally available for help. Your doctor's partners can be an important indicator of his or her values, and those doctors may, by default, be involved with your health care. Despite your best efforts to select your physician or specialist, that person you selected sometimes provides medical care that is only as good as his or her staff or the reciprocal relationships he or she has established with physicians on call.

The receptionist or nurse at your doctor's office will usually be your first line of communication. These individuals represent the office and the doctor, and the way they behave usually reflects the doctors who have hired them. If they are rude or impossible to reach on the telephone, this is clearly a negative sign, but don't be completely put off. If a doctor meets all of your other criteria, you must have a serious conversation with him or her regarding how the office staff treats you. In some instances, doctors may be unaware of how their employees deal with patients. Never allow office behavior to stop you from selecting the best doctor for you, but be sure you are clear with your physician about how you expect to be treated. The reverse is also true: When the office staff is kind and accommodating, you should go out of your way to thank them, make them feel special, and compliment them to the doctor they work for.

Usually you can gain the information you need about your doctor by being courteous, open, and respectful (but not passive). After all, those qualities are among those you will want to maintain with a physician, and a good one, from the beginning, will show them to you in kind.

Financial issues may interfere with the quality of your care.

This is particularly true when a physician is selling his practice. Although it is technically illegal for a doctor to sell access to his or her patients, it is quite common for an outgoing physician to steer patients to an incoming or nearby physician. The conflict of interest arises when the outgoing physician has a financial interest or partnership agreement for a percentage of the incoming physician's profits. It is always best to make your own evaluations in the event of your doctor's extended leave or retirement. And if you do seek your health care elsewhere, arrange to transfer or take copies of your medical records with you. You do have the legal right to obtain your records.

Many other conflicts of interest arise from financial inducements. The large drug and pharmaceutical companies lobby physicians to use their products. Companies quite commonly wine and dine physicians at expensive restaurants or offer rewards for prescribing a particular brand-name product. These incentives can lead to overreliance on a particular product, even if there are safer and better treatments available. Relationships between physicians and product salespeople are difficult for patients to investigate, but there are telltale signs. A stream of drug salespeople in the waiting room or exiting your physician's office with those annoying rolling briefcases can be a warning. Another thing I look for are notepads and pens with drug logos on them. Always ask your doctor what other choices exist for your ailment, and why he or she chose that particular one for you. You should also ask what percentage of his patients use the drug you are using, and how many are on the other possible medications.

The biggest problem is overprescription of drugs with multiplying side effects instead of encouragement toward alternative therapies. Before you begin a drug regime, ask your doctor what other medicines are available to treat your particular problem. Make certain that you clearly understand why he or she has chosen a particular drug for you and that you are aware of possible side effects or interactions with other medications and dietary supplements.

CASELOADS, CLEANLINESS, AND EQUIPMENT

A number of nonmedical factors are also important. The most significant is a physician's caseload. You should be able to get an appointment within a reasonable amount of time. Also consider the physician's secretary and other medical staff. If a doctor's staff is not accessible, knowledgeable, helpful, and friendly, the source is often the physician or office manager who hired them. You should not have trouble getting through to set up an appointment or to have a simple question answered.

Once you arrive at the office, you should not have to camp out in the waiting room for hours unless there is an unusual emergency situation that has been explained to you. Your doctor could be trying to save on the expense of taking on a partner, or perhaps is trying to crowd too many patients into his or her schedule, knowing that a certain number always cancel. Never be afraid to tell your doctor about difficulty in being able to reach him or her. You can evaluate his or her response and decide whether or not you feel that it is fair, realistic, and an answer you can live with.

Other key factors include the cleanliness of the physician's office and the personal and professional habits of the doctor and staff. Take note if the furniture is shabby or stained, or whether the examination room is poorly lighted. The appearance of the office may not directly affect the care that is given, but it can be a good indicator of a physician's priorities. Evan Levine, a prominent physician who has written candidly about the subject, always checks the kind of stethoscope a doctor is using. A top-of-the-line stethoscope costs less than two hundred dollars, yet you may be surprised how often some physicians will skimp on the premium item, despite its being one of the primary tools of their trade. Stethoscopes with pink tubing, or ones with a drug company logo on them, which cost in the neighborhood of five dollars, are sure signs that you are dealing with a doctor cutting costs at the expense of your good care.

THE SLIPPERY SLOPE OF SPECIALIST REFERRALS

Much the same criteria you used for selecting your PCP should be employed in choosing a specialist. Many patients rely entirely on their PCP to refer them to the specialists who will be part of their team. This is not necessarily a bad idea, and it can be an advantage. If you have built a relationship with your PCP, he or she is likely in the best position to know your needs and, moreover, to have observed that specialist in action. However, several very good reasons exist for not leaving the decision-making solely to your PCP. In many cases—far more than the medical establishment admits—physicians may not keep themselves abreast of the latest medical breakthroughs, and may not know which specialists are up-to-date on the advanced knowledge of their fields. The fault here, if you should encounter it knowingly or not, may not rest entirely with your PCP; the mass of new medical information released each year presents a daunting challenge for the general practitioner, especially one who graduated from medical school twenty to forty years ago.

In certain instances your PCP may have a conflict of interest in making recommendations, especially when that specialist is a partner in the same medical practice, or is the one your health plan wants your PCP to recommend, or is a personal friend. Therefore, it is important to ask exactly why your PCP has recommended a particular specialist. Ask if there are other specialists in this field and whether he would mind if you consulted one of them. If any doctor does not allow you to seek a second opinion, he or she is definitely the wrong doctor for you.

In this step, and virtually every one you take, it is important for you to become aware, educate yourself, and ask questions. At the very least you should understand the general process by which a physician becomes a specialist. In other words, you've got to know what that specialist is bringing to the table.

THE IMPORTANCE OF BEING UP-TO-DATE

The training of a specialist begins after the new M.D. begins what is called a residency. In years past, the first year of post–medical school training was called an internship, but the entire sequence is now called a residency. Resident physicians dedicate themselves for three to seven years or full-time experience in a hospital or health care setting in which they and other specialists in training care for patients under the supervision of an experienced physician in their field. Medical conferences and research projects are often part of that training. In choosing your specialists, it is vital to find out exactly what education and training he or she has completed. It is also essential to determine whether or not your doctor's clinic or medical group has a great reputation in the specialty you need.

The object of your research is to gauge the ability of your specialist to perform a given task. His or her bedside manner and willingness to get to know you personally may not figure into your decisions as prominently as with your PCP, but the same rules apply. The skill you will want in a surgeon is the ability to perform a procedure flawlessly. Being up-to-date on that procedure is of paramount importance, because protocols for these procedures change constantly.

As an example, recently my father-in-law was feeling oddly

winded when he exercised, so he went to a cardiologist at Columbia-Presbyterian, in New York City, who ordered an angiogram. He soon learned that five arteries to his heart had severe blockage. Not long ago a cardiologist would have routinely recommended immediate open-heart surgery and a quintuple bypass, an extremely high-risk operation with a very long recovery period. Instead, my father-in-law was given the newest and greatest option. Instead of undergoing open-heart surgery, he was treated with a new and highly successful procedure that is far less invasive and far less dangerous. While he was fairly conscious, stents were placed in all five arteries during two procedures; he recovered quickly and was discharged from the hospital within twenty-four hours. He is doing unbelievably well. Had he not gone to that particular doctor and that particular hospital, he might have faced an extremely risky operation and many long months of recuperation. Medical techniques are constantly evolving—you want the most skilled doctor who is both aware of the latest medical advances and able to perform them perfectly.

If you need surgery, always ask to be the first surgery of the day. The surgeon and the surgical team will be fresh and well rested then, and the operating room will be at its most sterile. The later your surgery is scheduled in the day, the more risk of a tired surgeon and tired surgical team. There is also a greater chance that you will experience delays of many hours, since incoming emergencies will have priority over scheduled procedures in the operating room. Normally you are required to fast from midnight the night before your operation, so the longer you have to wait, the more hungry, thirsty, anxious, and uncomfortable you become. When you are having surgery, the experience is frightening and nerve-racking, no matter how minor anyone tells you it will be. Remember the difference between minor surgery and major surgery: If it is happening to someone else, it is minor surgery; if it is happening to you, it is major surgery.

How do you find the best? In medical procedures, practice makes perfect. A surgeon who does not perform surgeries regularly may be out of practice—or dangerously out of touch with the latest advances. Of course you must consider variables. A surgeon needs the ability to make good decisions quickly and under pressure. Some operations take hours of concentration; others are short and routine. For most procedures, your surgeon should be performing two hundred surgeries a year to be up-to-date. The criteria for a neurologist might place great emphasis on technical knowledge, success rates, and years of experience.

Unfortunately, there is no federal regulatory group for physicians. Almost all certification and verification is done at the state level. Even at this level, public information is modest. As mentioned earlier, you can obtain information about a doctor's education and his certifications. However, few states provide data regarding numbers of procedures an individual doctor has performed. Thus, few hospitals keep such statistics. The best way to obtain and evaluate such information is to ask your doctor and then see if the hospital where he or she practices confirms the estimate. If such cold calculation seems insensitive to you, remember that you or someone you love is going under the knife. You have to be sure.

Regardless of his or her specialty, however, you want a specialist who will listen to your concerns and will respect your feelings and wishes. Think twice about a specialist whose attitude is "I'm the expert so do as I say." If a physician ignores your directives or simply moves you out of the office too quickly, declare that you are not satisfied with such care and consult someone else.

Be certain that surgery is definitely the only option. Ask your doctor if it may be possible to remedy the situation any other way. Surgery is expensive and some doctors look at surgeries as good business. There is a well-known phrase in the medical world: "A surgeon likes to cut." This means that surgery is what they have been trained to do—for them, it may well be the first option they consider, not the last. Make sure that they have considered other, less invasive alternatives before concluding that surgery is the best choice for you. Surgery always carries inherent risks.

Note, however, that if you decide to change specialists or surgeons (and, possibly, the hospitals they are attached to), the change can mean weeks or months of delay for tests or operations, especially when an HMO is involved. Find the specialist staff member and hospital administrators who can willingly and efficiently help make the change. Be persistent and positive, and you will find them. Never go under the knife of a doctor whom you do not fully trust.

CHECK BOARD CERTIFICATION

The best place to start researching prospective specialists is to learn whether they have been board certified in their field. Just because a doctor specializes or has earned a reputation for certain treatments does not guarantee that he or she has been tested or taken special training in that field. A board-certified physician has taken necessary additional study and must undergo periodic examinations to ensure that his or her knowledge is up-to-date. If the specialist is not board certified, it should be a warning. The American Board of Medical Specialists (toll-free, 866-275-2267) can give you this information. Another way to check on board certification is to visit the Internet site www.abms.org.

In choosing a specialist you will also want to consult statistical and legal records. Here again, be open to interpretation. In certain instances, a specialist may have an unblemished record because he or she accepts only low-risk patients who are in good health. Conversely, you might find, on inquiry, that the best surgeons actually have lower success rates. Patients in critical need have turned to them precisely because of their professional reputations and their willingness to risk their statistical standings for a patient's greater good.

Consider looking at teaching hospitals to find the specialist you need, but look with a critical eye. There, the experienced specialists who train medical residents are highly likely to be up on the latest cutting-edge technology and treatments. They perform hundreds more procedures than do physicians in smaller facilities. On the other hand, in many teaching hospitals it is not uncommon for a licensed resident to perform all or part of a procedure under the specialist's supervision. You may believe that you are getting a particular specialist's expertise when in fact you will receive only their supervision of your case. Very often, your surgeon might do the surgery and allow an associate to stitch up your incision. Stitches and staples that are not carefully placed can leave unattractive scars that you will not see until it is too late to correct. Insist on knowing who will be conducting all facets of your procedure.

Another good reason to consider consulting specialists at teaching hospitals or large medical centers is the cost of specialized treatment—it can, in many cases, be prohibitive, especially if a person doesn't have insurance or Medicaid. Most large teaching hospitals and medical centers have clinic systems or centers that provide some form of discounted care. These are staffed by physicians in training who are supervised by attending board-certified specialists. You may not get the particular physician you selected, but you are almost guaranteed superior treatment, sometimes better than if you paid thousands of dollars at a community hospital that is not as well staffed. If there is no teaching hospital in your area, in most cases one can be reached within an hour or two. Where your health is at stake, the travel is obviously worthwhile.

THE VALUE OF A SECOND OPINION

Regardless of whom you ultimately select to have on your medical team, it is still important to get second opinions from other doctors—no matter how satisfied you are with your physician, his or her diagnosis, and recommended treatment plan. No two doctors' opinions are exactly the same, even if they are the most brilliant and qualified physicians in their fields. It is not worth the risk when your life is on the line. At the very least, hearing different opinions will be a learning experience, as you gain knowledge and insight for decisions you need to make later on down the line.

Most important, ask questions. Your PCP, like your specialists, works for you, not the other way around. Nothing that concerns your interests is unimportant. You're entitled to know what's happening in your body, and the physicians you choose are a major source of your information.

HERE ARE SOME KEY QUESTIONS you will want to ask yourself:

- Does my doctor truly listen to what I'm trying to say? Does he or she let me communicate all my thoughts?
- Do I feel comfortable in his or her presence?
- Am I being treated courteously and with respect?
- Have all my questions been answered?

Here are some key questions you will want to ask your medical team:

- Are all the treatments that have been offered to me standard for my illness, or are new clinical-trial treatments available?
- What can I expect the outcome of my treatment to be? How quickly can I expect results? What results have other patients had?
- Are there other treatment options? What kinds of results have they given for patients?
- What are the side effects of the treatments suggested?
- Which drugs will a physician prescribe? How will they help me and what are their side effects?
- How will the drugs and treatments affect me on a day-to-day basis? Will I be able to work?
- If I have questions between visits, how do I reach the physician? What time of day is best? Does he or she generally return calls? Will the emergency phone number route me to an answering machine or to a living person?

Do not rely on your memory to absorb the information that your physician gives you. Carry a notepad or a journal and write down his or her comments. Better, ask your physician to write the information down for you. Many will do so without being asked. You may also tape-record your physician's advice. Make sure that your physician understands your desire to record his or her recommendations. Make any of these options part of your routine. If a physician can't give you adequate answers to your questions, or you want to know more, ask where you can get it. Also, ask whether your physician keeps a list of patient organizations for people with your condition.

Always remember: The doctor is working for *you*. This is your body. You are entitled to know what the doctor thinks— and why he or she has reached a particular conclusion about your condition, and what the treatment that he or she recommends for your health is based upon.

Step Four Summary

1. Begin your search for Dr. Right with your most trusted sources of recommendation: your friends and family.
2. Ask others in the medical profession—doctors and nurses—for their comments or suggestions about both primary care physicians and specialists.
3. Do your homework in the library and on the Internet to obtain information on the prospective doctor's training and professional experience.
4. Ask to meet your doctor's staff and colleagues who may be substituting when he or she is not available.
5. Observe how a prospective Dr. Right treats his or her staff, keeps the office, and reflects his or her values.
6. Check all of your doctors for board certification and lawsuits.
7. No matter how much you trust Dr. Right, always get a second opinion on any serious medical issue.

STEP FIVE

Build Your Health Team

FROM THE START OF THIS BOOK, I have emphasized how important it is to take total and unconditional responsibility for every aspect of your life: You must make decisions that encourage good health and happiness, must be your own best health care advocate, and must create the life you want. There is no getting around that truth.

It is also the truth that you can't possibly do it alone. You should not be expected to carry the entire burden and the flood of negative emotions yourself. This is especially true for a person who has been diagnosed with a chronic illness. Early in your recovery process you need to identify and build a positive support system for yourself. The sooner you do it, the better off you will be. It's important to get prepared for the various steps in your recovery so that you can have the most harmonious and fulfilling life possible from this moment on—and to do that you need help from the most optimistic, caring, and organized people you know.

YOUR HEALTH, INC
Your Name
CEO
The head of your very own health organization

COO
Your Health Care Advocate &
Right-Hand Person

Other Health Helpers
Nutritionist
Personal Trainer
Pharmacy Liaison

Administrative Aide
Communications Center

Director of Human Resources

Comfort Giver
Psychological & Spiritual Services

Domestic Assistance
Housekeeper
Child Care
Driver
Cook

CFO
Your Financial Nerve Center
from Insurance to Legal Matters

Lawyer

You may or may not be ready, willing, and able to manage everyday things like getting out of bed, bathing, dressing, and preparing meals. You may or may not need someone to help clean the house or shop for groceries. On the other hand, you may find that delegating some of these chores and responsibilities will give you more time to tackle your primary goal.

A NEW JOB DESCRIPTION: CEO OF YHI

From the moment that you were diagnosed, you were given a new set of goals and responsibilities. Some people find it easier to understand this life adjustment as a new job assignment. You have been appointed chief executive officer (CEO) of Your Health, Inc. This is a large and important position, the most important in your life. Everything else in your life must be either set aside or given a role in Your Health. Friends and family must understand that either they are on your "wellness bus" in some supportive way, or they simply are standing by the roadside to watch this part of your life journey.

Your wellness is a project to be managed, and the best way to manage it is to find the best help available. When you assemble the right team for Your Health, Inc., you will be able to concentrate on being well and to avoid the extra stress that always attends illness. I have sketched out a system whereby you can classify the kind of help you need. I have also provided some tips about how to search for and recruit that help—whether it's from your family, close friends, fellow employees, clergy, or paid helpers. Once you have identified them, there is a suggested organizational plan to coordinate everyone's efforts.

Please understand that the team concept and the job descriptions that you will read are the ultimate dream team. Not everybody can command the small army I am suggesting. However, the value in presenting the ideal structure with descriptions of positions is that you can see the whole picture and can tailor the ideal structure to the realities of your needs and resources. Your efforts to seek assistance in those areas of your life will be rewarded later on.

Because chronic illness strikes people differently, you undoubtedly will want to tailor any plan to your own needs. Depending on your creativity, your network of family and friends, and your financial comfort level, you may come up with additional ways that I have not suggested to accommodate the support work. Each situation will be different, but it helps to start with a blueprint. You can avoid some of the early uncertainties I had by taking advantage of this system.

∞

NONE OF THIS IS EASY. When I woke up the day after my diagnosis, I was unprepared for the flood of information I was to be given and the many decisions I had to make in a very short period of time. I was in a fog—a common occurrence, I've learned, when people receive a life-altering or life-threatening diagnosis. Fortunately, many people came to my aid. They were on hand to help with the long stream of X-rays, CAT scans, MRIs, and other diagnostic testing I was to undergo. Since my very first crisis, I had help from my parents and friends. They helped me assimilate and understand the barrage of information coming at me and enabled me to make reasonable and sane decisions about my health care. In the process I learned—and I think you will, too—who really cared for me and who didn't. It was the beginning of a major change in my life, and that change was for the better. I never knew I was worthy of that much love from anybody. It made me feel truly great in ways I had never felt before.

BUILDING A SUPPORT TEAM IS A SIGN OF STRENGTH

The ability to delegate activities yet stay in control of your life is a powerful skill, a strength that should be applauded. Some people misunderstand the concept of a support team and believe that it means giving up control over aspects of your life to others. Nothing could be further from the truth. If you do it well, which may not be easy, you will be able to accomplish all of the tasks that you have always done and then focus on every aspect of your health. For some, such leadership comes naturally; for others, it must be learned. You do not have a choice in this matter. You must ask for and accept the help of others in this crisis, so that you can concentrate on finding the path back to health. The better you can guide others and allow them to help you, the more you can accomplish toward your wellness. Don't be afraid of making some mistakes along the way. It is only natural to do so. Those mistakes will help you make future judgments about what is right for you. Later, you will reach the point when you have regained your strength and your health with the help of others. Then, it is time for you to help others. You will feel the ultimate reward.

∞

As CHIEF EXECUTIVE OFFICER of Your Health, Inc., you are at the center of the project for your well-being. Your first duty is to find the very best people to work on your team. Below is a general description of some roles that need to be filled in any wellness campaign; you may need to add others or to alter some of the job descriptions. These jobs can be combined in different ways, but each designation, clearly defined by you, will move you forward in your search for your perfect health-advocacy team.

Where do you start? A good way to begin is with that time-tested tool: a list. List the tasks your team will need to perform. Then, make a list of the friends, family, neighbors, or co-workers who may be willing to help. Once you have linked some names with some tasks, you can assess who might become the best overall health advocate on your team. That person may serve a dual role, or he or she may serve primarily as a liaison between you and your doctors, providing background information and advice, to the exclusion of other responsibilities for your care.

YOUR HEALTH ADVOCATE

Ideally, your advocate is your alter ego. This is the person who will share your most intimate secrets and who will have the greatest responsibility for decisions about your health—other than yourself. This is the person you will want at your side if you have to go to the emergency room or if you have to be admitted to the hospital. He or she will also coordinate the search for information and help you study your disease.

It is a tough job. This person must be able to keep you thinking positively—sometimes even very good friends are not emotionally capable of taking on the advocate role because of their personal sadness about your diagnosis. No matter how close these friends or family members are to you, if all they can offer is gloom and doom, you must not let them assume this position. Your health advocate is the person who will in effect be you, even to the extent of making the legal and medical choices you would make for yourself when and if you are unable to do so.

In a corporate structure, your advocate would be the chief operating officer, your number two, your most valued adviser, and your likely successor. You need someone close to you—someone with an overview, someone with enough time to devote to you in your time of need—to be with you when you confer with doctors, technicians, and clerks. This person has done some medical research with you and knows what to expect. When you are very ill you don't always comprehend or process what your doctor is saying. Your advocate should be able to hear and understand the information your doctor has conveyed—and if necessary interpret it for you and ask questions for clarification. Your health care advocate should help you to fill out and to understand every single medical fact about you on your Very Necessary Medical Identification Card (see page 249). The word *advocate* is both a noun and a verb. He or she should be able to convey your wishes—to champion your health decisions and to be your health advocate in every sense. Your ideal health advocate should be both loyal support (the noun) and ready to move or to speak on your behalf (the verb). Remember: This can be one person or a team of many.

YOUR HEALTH ADVOCATE VS. HOSPITAL PATIENT ADVOCATE

Many people think personal health advocates and hospital patient advocates are the same. They are not. The latter designation belongs to the hospital's ombudsman for patients' rights. He or she is appointed by the hospital or health center to address a patient's unique problems or complaints while in its care. A patient advocate can be very helpful and kind; however, never forget that he or she is ultimately responsible to the institution, not to you personally. Even after your hospital stay is over, you will still need an advocate to work with you on your long-term care and recovery.

CHOOSING AN ADVOCATE

Those closest to you are the first people to whom you will turn to find an advocate. Your spouse or significant other may seem the most logical choice, but some will find, as I did, that he or she may not be able to fulfill that duty. Your partner may be overwhelmed, overly emotional, overloaded by all of your mutual responsibilities, or just in denial. As difficult as it will be, you must make careful, reasoned judgments about everyone on your team—and especially about your advocate. Many people may be important parts of your life and may be able to offer love and support. However, your advocate is crucial.

In your interviews with advocate candidates, you must speak freely and candidly. The two of you are going to need completely honest communication in the future and you must begin on that basis. How your prospective advocate reacts to sensitive subjects about your care and treatment is a good indicator of whether he or she is the right person to head your team. A highly emotional response—such as anguish and tears—may be a sign of how much someone cares about you, but it is not an indication of the clearheaded and calm person who is to be the captain of your ship in the middle of this storm.

The health care advocate you choose will be closely linked to the team you have assembled to look out for your interests. The challenge is not to anticipate all possible scenarios or situations that might come along. You and your advocate must encourage a dynamic that is supportive and understanding of individual team members' needs and desires. The two of you will strive to build around you a structure that will make it easy to delegate responsibilities and handle whatever concerns arise. Write down your needs, ask particular individuals to help with certain responsibilities, and clearly explain and discuss what you would like them to do.

Being an advocate is a momentous and time-consuming responsibility, and you may find that one individual doesn't always have enough free time to be your advocate in all situations. You may also discover that some people close to you deal better with some issues than they do with others. In both of these instances, consider assembling a team of medical advocates who work well together. In this and in all other matters, the key is communication.

Just as you have sought to educate yourself to understand medical jargon, so must your advocate. Your spouse or best friend may be a good candidate, but a friend or relative who is a nurse, a medical technician, or even a medical secretary may prove more effective because their learning curve will not be as steep. Your trust is important, of course, as are an advocate's intuition and common sense. Equally important, however, is that the person understands what is taking place from a medical standpoint and knows the importance of making appropriate decisions in the most timely way. Knowledge of the medical reality of your condition in a life-or-death situation can help steer the outcome to life.

I have already written about the extraordinary support I received from my parents. They remain my ideal role models for a set of health advocates. My mom provided my emotional sustenance and saw to it that I got the best doctors everywhere. She also took care of my kids when I went out of town to seek medical opinions. Dad supervised the technical aspects, conferring with doctors and making sure that I got the best possible care. Even before that, of course, he had already led by example, showing me by his own experience how to confront a challenging diagnosis. They will always be my superheroes!

I am so thankful for my friends, who also played a very important role as health advocates. Lynn Palmer, Brenda Richie, and Kathryn Belton came with me for that Sunday MRI, when we all first learned that I had a serious problem. Together with my forever friends, Debbie and Jimmy Lustig from Denver, they helped me emotionally, hugged me and cried with me, and they helped my young sons deal with my health issues, as they are also their godparents. They felt sorry for me, then quickly got out of the pity mode to help me fight for the best possible outcome. They did research, sent flowers and cards, accompanied me to appointments, and with their positive outlook pushed me to make my way out of the negative emotional mind-set that came with my "no hope—go home—go to bed" prognosis. My sister, Dana Davis, who is so strong and courageous with her diabetes, offered this important advice to me about accepting MS: "At least you know what you have so you can truly deal with it." Many people aren't so lucky as they have a mystery illness with no real direction to follow.

And that was just the beginning. To this day, they have all remained my closest confidants. They have been very important in my MS care and other medical crises, such as losing my baby, having surgery, and then the ultimate joy of having my blessed twin baby girls. They and so many other family and friends, such as my caring and supportive brothers, John and Gregg Davis, who gave me a great shoulder to lean on late at night when things got depressing, Pam McMahon, Jo Champa, Tawny Sanders, and Tracy and Tony Danza, have been on my side. Together with my mother, Tom Arnold, Tommy Hilfiger, and Natalie Cole, they have continued to champion my cause, working endless hours to help raise money for multiple sclerosis research and for my yearly RACE to Erase MS event. By giving me such a positive outlook on life, they have encouraged my good health, and I know that if I ever have another health problem or they do, we have grown through one another's crises to be a group who would truly support one another no matter what. They are all part of this complicated jigsaw puzzle put together as one that equals life.

WHAT SKILLS SHOULD ADVOCATES HAVE in order to do a good job for you, while remaining stress-free themselves? The poet Rudyard Kipling expressed one attribute eloquently:

> *If you can keep your head when all about you*
> *Are losing theirs and blaming it on you,*
> *If you can trust yourself when all men doubt you,*
> *But make allowance for their doubting too . . .*
> *Yours is the Earth and everything that's in it . . .*

Let's look at a few of the other qualities you need to consider when looking for an advocate:

- **Affability:** He or she should be willing to become your counselor, researcher, and perhaps even treatment administrator and monitor. If your medical team has not yet been selected, your advocate may help you locate and evaluate the best doctor based on your individual needs. He or she should expect to communicate with your medical team on your behalf whenever necessary. Having good relationships with other members of your support team constitutes another "plus" quality for your ideal advocate.

- **Availability:** This seems an obvious item, but it requires some thought. If a person close to you is willing to help as an advocate but works two jobs—or has two small children—it is unlikely that he or she will have the time to race to the hospital if necessary or go with you to important meetings with your providers. This is why sometimes it is important to have a team of advocates. You never want to spend time in a hospital without an advocate to monitor your nursing care and to make sure that your meds are correct and administered on time. Also, he or she must be sure you are not given anything that you may be allergic to. If your partner cannot do it, then who can? Often, someone you least expect will step up and volunteer. That's what I mean by knowing who your friends are and what their limitations are.

- **Confidentiality:** You may require that your health advocate make medical decisions either with you or on your behalf. If that is an eventuality, you need to know that you can trust him or her with intimate information. If you have confidence in your advocate's ability and confidentiality, you may wish to provide that individual with a durable power of attorney or to set up a living trust that will be administered by the person you select. One of the most delicate subjects we face today entails permissions for or prohibitions against life support in the event of a coma or inability to convey one's own wishes. You may want to donate your organs, as I have requested to be done upon my death. All these wishes should be documented in writing, with your custodian clearly identified. An advocate can help in securing these important papers.

- **Experience:** Ideally, the person you choose should have some medical experience in order to understand the complexities of your treatment. He or she should expect to collect information from your doctor, coordinate with the other members of your team, and participate knowledgeably in discussions about your treatment. If you are on a steep learning curve when first diagnosed with MS, as I was, your advocate should be willing to plunge in and take on the task of compiling your questions. Your advocate must write things down when you cannot and help you find answers and do research, as well as confer with health care professionals about your alternatives.

- **Diplomacy:** Obviously, you want someone to help you who will not unnecessarily upset you, your friends, or the medical team you have assembled. The ideal advocate can give information without becoming imperious, and take it in without being too emotional. At the same time, you need someone who is not afraid to speak up when there is a need. Am I asking you to find a saint? No. But it is in your best interest to look for someone who has the ability and the will to encourage a supportive dynamic among all your team members.

JOB DESCRIPTIONS FOR THE REST OF THE SUPPORT TEAM

Without a doubt, your advocate is the most important person on your support team, which is why I have examined the job qualifications in such detail. Without going into as many specifics, let us consider the job descriptions for the rest of your team. As you think about these roles, consider that more than one person, helping on a revolving basis, may be needed to fill one job. Conversely, a single dedicated helper may be able to help you in more than one area or even in all areas.

Health Care Financial Administrator

Unfortunately, as a person with a chronic illness, you will hear many people in the health care business yelling, "Show me the money!" Doctors, nurses, specialists, hospitals, ambulance ser-vices, laboratories, departments that deal with MRIs, EKGs, sonography, radiography, and many other specialties will all be providing you with help—at a price. Later in this book we will

explore how to contain these costs (see Step Nine: "Tame the
Health Care Monster"). For now, you need to know how to select a person to control the flow of paper and set up a dedicated
file system for the finances of Your Health, Inc.

In a corporate structure, that person would be your chief financial officer. Ideally, he or she should have some knowledge
of medical billing and coding. Health care providers and insurers literally have a language, a system of codes, and a way of
dealing with billing and payment that is unique to the medical
system. You need a person who already knows some of these
functions or is willing to spend the time to figure them out.

Your accountant may be a whiz when it comes to the Internal Revenue Service and the world of investments, but medical
finance is a different story. It would be natural to think that
someone who is familiar with your regular financial affairs
might be the right person to handle this important area for Your
Health, Inc., but this is much more than a numbers-crunching
position. Your CFO must have a grasp of the structure of the
health care business and an understanding of the complex financial relationships between providers and insurers. He or she
must be prepared to speak the language of health care and to go
to bat for you, if need be. Insurers frequently deny benefits and
refuse to pay doctors and labs—even when you are clearly entitled to coverage. It will take a firm and persistent individual
who is prepared to deal with your insurer on the phone—repeatedly, if necessary—to make sure you are getting the benefits
to which you are entitled.

If you have friends—or even friends of friends—who have
some of this specialized financial knowledge and are willing to
help you, accept this blessing. Otherwise, closely question potential candidates who have financial experience outside of the
medical world. There is simply no way that they can help you
without dedicating considerable effort to learn about the

health care system. In a perfect world, your CFO would analyze bills and keep records that were far more detailed and complicated than any he or she had ever seen before. This may not be possible for everyone. If you can afford it, hire accountants with the specialized knowledge or consultants who will guide you through the maze. If, understandably, you cannot afford such specialized help, try to find someone who can help you keep the papers organized. You may be able to get some assistance from either the hospital office or your doctor's office.

Do not be lulled into a complacent attitude about this just because you and your doctor have dealt with some medical bills before. I do not intend to frighten you; rather, I want to make you aware so that you can manage this important area. The billings for a chronic illness can quickly become a mountain of bewildering facts and figures. Even with good health insurance, the costs can escalate and the paperwork can get out of hand. Be prepared. Be knowledgeable. Have a financial administrator ready to help you through your recovery. Please do not end up healthy but bankrupt, as some people have.

Health Care Administrative Aide

In the old, politically incorrect days, the person who held this job in a corporation was called an executive secretary, and the dirty little secret of most boardrooms was that these people (most of them women) were the executives' brains. This individual is the organizer, the person who knows the names of your children's teachers, the telephone numbers where they can be reached, and probably their schedules. This is the person who knows the name of the person at the front desk in your doctor's office, the one who can find a copy of the prescription your specialist gave you two weeks ago, along with the notes from your advocate who translated your doctor's explanation of what this drug does. The organizer maintains the complete and current list of your support team's home phone and cell phone numbers, e-mail addresses, and schedules.

In an ideal world, this person would be your administrative assistant who recently retired and is willing to step in to help you. Most likely this would be your spouse, secretary, or best friend. You need someone who is well organized, accustomed to keeping records, and comfortable with keeping schedules, working lines of communication, and finding important data when you need it. Presumably, he or she would work closely with you, your advocate, and your financial administrator to maintain vital information and to communicate with both your medical personnel and your support team.

Your administrative aide should also be the keeper of the paper trail. State laws usually require that patients be given copies of their complete medical records, and you will want to have all of yours. You will need a filing system for medical records, tests, insurance letters, and notes of meetings. If nothing else, it is important to have someone keep track of the maze of insurance interactions you will undoubtedly encounter. If you have a clear record of your meetings, letters, and other interactions with your doctor's billing office, hospitals, and health care insurers, your financial administrator will be in a much stronger position to contain the costs, pay the bills, and, if necessary, do battle with your insurance company.

Your aide may prepare your correspondence, make written requests for records, coordinate with consulting physicians, and organize the copies of records you may need to take to your appointments. He or she should also keep track of personal health-care record keeping. The aide should make a log of appointment dates, reasons for the visit, and doctor's name and location. He or she should establish files for diagnosis and treatment instructions, questions asked and answered, and baseline information like blood pressure. He or she must know which medicines you are taking and which ones would be detrimental to your health.

As if this multitasking administrative aide did not have enough to do, he or she may also take on the role of communications central. This person may be the one who contacts all family members and friends to update them on your condition.

Lawyer

Most people don't think about legal services until they are needed. However, there are a number of reputable attorneys who provide "insurance policies" for legal affairs. A yearly retainer provides you with a certain level of service for legal transactions possibly including drawing up living wills, setting up living trusts and finding conservators—even representing you in legal discussions with insurance companies.

A single meeting with an attorney can uncover which alternatives are available. Living trusts, in particular, are valuable tools for clearly stating your desires about your welfare and that of your family. An attorney will know how to place this information in a document that is legally binding and in accord with the laws of your state. You may designate who will care for your children, who will have authority to write checks for you, and whether you want to be attached to a respirator or receive blood or drugs such as morphine. A lawyer should help you and your advocate to prepare any necessary documents. Important basic forms are available through the Legal Counsel for the Elderly (www.aarp.org/lce/ or www .uaelderlaw.org) a service of the American Association of Retired Persons (AARP).

When people become ill, they are often in denial and cannot face the possibility of their mortality. In reality, it is of the utmost importance to draw up a will so that you can properly take care of your family if you don't survive. If you ignore this, your assets will not go where you would want them to. Instead, they could go to the government.

In most cases, your family lawyer can handle health care issues for you. If you anticipate more complications, contact a legal specialist—perhaps by recommendation from your family lawyer—about a retainer or "insurance relationship."

Pharmacy Liaison

Assign one person to order and maintain your medicines and other supplies that you need on a regular basis. If that one person becomes familiar with your vendors and pharmacists, it will be easier to order and receive emergency items quickly. He or she will also become knowledgeable about your medications, their interactions, and other pharmaceutical information. Needless to say, this is a person who will work closely with you and your advocate. If at all possible, try to use only one pharmacy for all of your medicines. This way, you can be assured that with the many different doctors you may be using, your prescriptions will not counteract each other and cause yet another medical emergency. Also, the pharmacy will keep your insurance papers on hand, which will expedite the filling of your prescriptions.

Director of Human Resources

There will be emotional issues that arise for almost every member of your family and support team. You cannot deal with all of them, nor can your advocate. You need a buffer who can deal with the day-to-day problems that are inevitable. Any illness— whether sudden or chronic—can wreak havoc on a family.

When one family member is diagnosed with a disease, it is as if the whole family has the disease—and every side effect that comes with it. Immediately, relationships are threatened, level heads become unpredictable, and daily routines turn upside down. At such times, it is desirable to find someone who can promote calm and quiescence. As I've already pointed out, you can't do it all alone. This person may be able to keep your support team running smoothly and to obtain the services of a psychological or spiritual counselor, should such help be necessary.

Other Health Care Helpers

There are many possibilities for nonmedical personnel to be a part of your support team. A healing diet is vital to your health, and periodic consultations with a nutritionist may be helpful. If you require a special program of exercise, the services of a physical therapist or a personal trainer who will come to the house may facilitate a significant aspect of your health regime. Depending on your circumstances, you may need a driver to take you to doctors' appointments, to hospitals or clinics for testing or medical procedures, or to physical therapy sessions.

Domestic Assistance

You and your spouse or life partner may have very strong feelings about privacy and domestic responsibility. Under normal circumstances, this is admirable. However, the diagnosis of a life-threatening or life-altering disease changes your situation—at least through the period of your recovery. You need to focus your energy on *your health*. This may mean allowing someone to help you with the preparation of meals or shopping. This may also mean that someone will help you with housekeeping, cleaning, laundry, and other domestic chores.

Even more sensitive is the issue of child care. This is an especially hard time for children of any age, and they need so much extra kindness and reassurance. Depending on the ages and circumstances of your children, you may wish to consult a child psychologist for advice on how to help them to deal with your health issues. During this period, older children are more likely to understand that you need your time and energy to fight a disease; this can be part of their contribution to your recovery. Younger children may require a different approach, including the closer involvement of grandparents or friends. Even the logistics can be a challenge—trustworthy people who will drive your children to school and pick them up from school or from lessons can make a huge contribution to your health team. Friends who are willing to help with homework or share family time can also be an important support. Allow friends and family to help you with simple but time-consuming tasks. You have a big job of your own.

Comfort Givers

I have already written about the damage that stress can do to your immune system and your general health. In addition to having a support team that will help you in many stressful areas of your life, you will profit from having friends or family who want simply to dedicate some time to your relaxation and comfort. This could be as simple as a friend who will bring a DVD or take you to the movies. Depending on your situation, you may need someone to read newspapers or books to you. You may prefer a friend who will just take a walk with you or chat on the phone. Simple pleasures that we take for granted become more difficult with chronic illness, but, awkward as it may seem, they are worth planning.

A NETWORK OF HUMAN BONDS

Your Health, Inc., your corporation for wellness, may prove to be the most heartwarming part of your journey. There are many ways to find the support you need. People within your religious community or hospital or hospice volunteers can come to your aid. The friends you already have and the ones you make through this support team will leave an indelible network of human bonds that both honor and celebrate your life, as well as enrich theirs. I know that I have gained immeasurably from the friendships developed by working with my support team. My mother, husband, children, brothers and sister, and the greatest friends in history have meant everything in my getting and staying healthy. They are constantly there and have given so unselfishly that I have learned a whole new appreciation for the human spirit.

That is what I wish for you—the life of a "normal citizen," surrounded by people who are willing to help. Sometimes we need to compensate professionals for their time; sometimes we find help from social or religious services; but most of the time, we have friends and supporters we never imagined.

The first step is to open yourself enough to say the words, "I need your help."

(Perhaps more than any other step in this process, the creation of a health care team may seem overwhelming. As I have stated repeatedly, having all of these team members will not be possible for everyone. What I have presented is the ideal. However, you need to know the entire picture so that you can deal with as many of the inevitable problems as possible. This will not happen overnight. It may take years to decide how to cope with all of the aspects of your new life. It took me many years to put together both the people and the procedures that make my health care more efficient and effective.)

Step Five Summary

1. Think of yourself as chief executive officer of Your Health, Inc.
2. Consider the ideal health care team; then, tailor your resources to meet your reality.
3. Learn one of the most important principles of leadership: how to delegate.
4. Designate a health advocate—a person who can step in to fill your shoes if needed and will be your most knowledgeable and avid supporter under all circumstances.
5. Be sure that your health advocate is kept as well informed and as up-to-date on all information regarding your health as you are.
6. Find a personal health-care financial administrator—a person who knows, or is willing to learn, the world of medical finance, and who is willing to keep track of the money in your case.
7. Find a health care administrative aide—a communicator, scheduler, and record keeper who can be a traffic cop for the entire team and a second brain for you, in order to keep this important organization running smoothly.
8. Depending on your situation, you may need legal services, domestic assistance, child care, family liaisons, or many other forms of help.
9. Lean on others. Enjoy and encourage the friendships that you develop with the people who share their abilities to support you in your time of need. Always thank them and show your gratitude.

STEP SIX

You Are What You Ingest

A HEALING DIET will make all of your other health efforts more effective. These changes in your eating habits are also the least difficult step in your journey to good health. Put simply, you must do everything you can to eliminate unhealthful foods and other substances that may have contributed to your illness in the first place. Then you must provide your body with the nutrients to repair, rebuild, cleanse, and energize itself. In my case, and for many other people who have a chronic condition, making informed decisions about diet has been the most important way to regain health. This includes giving up toxins you may consume in the form of alcohol, tobacco, nonprescription drugs, illegal drugs, or anything else you ingest.

THIS IS NOT THE TIME TO KID YOURSELF

Addictive substances such as alcohol and tobacco—and obviously drugs like cocaine, Ecstasy, and OxyContin—are dangerous even for healthy people to put into their systems. If you have a life-altering or life-threatening disease, it is a fact that these substances will make your disease accelerate. If you have this book in your hands, you are an intelligent person who is ready to be proactive in fighting your disease and restoring yourself to health. Do not kid yourself about your addictions. You have to be completely honest and stop using these substances immediately, if you can. If you can't do it on your own, get help—find a twelve-step program, substance-abuse counselor, or a rehab center. Get a sponsor and do everything you possibly can to kick your habit. It will never be easier to quit: your life is at stake.

If you are using over-the-counter painkillers or other non-prescription drugs or supplements, tell your doctor about them. Give yourself a chance: don't poison yourself. You must share information with your doctor about everything you are putting into your body, from aspirin to vitamins to muscle relaxers. Many people lie to themselves and go to a multitude of doctors for a variety of ailments. They get numerous medications from their physicians, but never report to each doctor the medications they are getting from the other MDs. This could be the sole reason for your illness. Many drugs are not effective when taken in combination with other medications. Others are downright toxic. Even vitamins, minerals, and herbal supplements can interact badly with certain medications. Talk to your doctor about possible drug interactions, but do your own homework as well. You should own a PDR (*Physician's Desk Reference*) and consult it before taking any newly prescribed drug.

My young friend Sally was diagnosed with MS, but "couldn't" stop smoking. Despite excellent medical advice and treatment, her condition deteriorated—and she continued to smoke. She knew that smoking played a part in lung cancer and heart disease, but she didn't believe that tobacco had been clinically connected to MS. She tried every MS drug but complained endlessly about how bad they all were and how depressed she was. Because Sally badly needed to strengthen her immune system, I begged her and warned her not to put poison into her body at such a crucial time. Sadly, she did not stop, and always blamed her bad health on everything but her smoking habit. She could never bring herself to take an honest look in the mirror and understand that none of the therapies had a chance of working while she was still addicted to nicotine. I believe that smoking was a major factor that eventually made her lose the battle.

You must give yourself the best chance possible to be healthy. You may feel that there is temporary solace in that cigarette or that glass of wine or that painkiller, but the cost is too high. When you are fighting for recovery, your system is fragile and needs all the help it can get to combat your disease. Don't kid yourself that putting more toxins into your system will help, or even that they will do no harm.

AN INCENTIVE FROM YOUR HEALTH INSURER

Health insurance companies take a dim view of addictive behaviors. As smokers are aware, they already pay higher premiums in many health care systems. Drinkers and drug abusers may not be aware that it is a fairly standard industry practice to consider you uninsurable for seven to ten years *after* you graduate from a rehab center or an addiction program. (In some cases, insurance may be issued with waivers at an extraordinarily high rate.)

Your goal is to become as knowledgeable as you can about your dietary needs and your body chemistry. Do not just rely on hearsay, or on the eating habits of your friends, whose nutri-

tional requirements may be very different from your own. Do
your homework. Study the relationship between good health
and nutrition. If you need to, consult a nutrition expert. The
food you eat must work for you and provide your body with the
building blocks of health. I think you will be surprised by how
appetizing and enjoyable the variety of foods in a healthy, healing diet can be. Never go on an extreme or faddish diet just to
lose weight. Such a diet may jeopardize your overall health by
lowering your immune system, which makes you more suscepti-
ble to diseases. Unless your doctor has a specific reason for rec-
ommending otherwise, you need a balanced diet that includes
protein, vegetables, fruits, fats, and grains in order to restore
and then maintain your health.

FIND THE RIGHT NUTRITION PLAN

There is an enormous number of diet and nutrition books available; it has never been easier to get the basic information you
need to get started. The challenge is to navigate those many resources to determine a nutrition plan that is right for you. As
you will discover, this process can be confusing, both because of
the volume of information available and because seemingly
knowledgeable dietary experts often contradict one another.
The team approach is best: consult and gain the support of your
physician and your health care team. Even if they are initially
uncertain about new and different approaches, the dialogue
will contribute to your collection of information. At the very
least, making even slight modifications in your diet can increase energy, improve mental alertness, relieve stress, and enhance the effectiveness of your treatment plan.

THIS IS NOT ABOUT LOSING —
OR GAINING — WEIGHT

The word *diet* has developed a contemporary connotation related to weight loss, bodybuilding, or medical restrictions. None of those areas is addressed in this chapter. You need to understand the importance of everything you put into your mouth. This chapter is about foods that will sustain health. I have consulted sources that base their information on clinical tests and medical surveys. I do not endorse any particular regime or restriction. I simply want you to know what the Mayo Clinic and the Harvard Medical School have learned about the healing values in various foods. (You may have heard about a "Mayo Clinic Diet," which has been denounced by the Mayo Clinic as a fraud. However, the Mayo Clinic has recently released a book setting forth its own healthy-eating principles, which focus on lots of fruits and vegetables.)

If you wish to conduct further research in this area, here are some useful references for discussion with your physician. *Eat, Drink, and Be Healthy: The Harvard Medical School Guide to Healthy Eating*, by Walter C. Willett, M.D., Ph.D., who is chairman of the Department of Nutrition at the Harvard School of Public Health and a Professor of Medicine at the Harvard Medical School, is a reliable guide. (This book also contains recipes, as well as an extensive section on suggested further reading about specific health/nutrition topics.) I have learned much from *Clinical Bioenergetics* (International Academy of Modern Bioenergetics), by Michael Galitzer, M.D., who has been one of my most helpful doctors in the field of nutrition. Updated health information can be found at www.mayoclinic.com.

ALWAYS CONSULT YOUR DOCTOR

Regardless of the information you may find in books and Internet sites, you must consult your physician about your diet. One person's condition will not be the same as another's, nor will one person respond to dietary changes as will another. It is important for you to know how your overall treatment plan is affected by what you eat and drink, including any supplements you may take. If you've ever been warned not to consume dairy products while taking antibiotics, you are already aware that foods can have chemical interactions with pharmaceuticals. It is essential that you inform your doctor of your dietary plan; he or she in turn can alert you to possible interaction problems. Taking certain medicines might even build up a food allergy that you had never experienced previously. The more knowledgeable you become, the more quickly you can incorporate what you have learned into your diet.

As you investigate and research, expect to find conflicting information. The world of nutrition is full of controversy. Major disagreements still exist among experts on big questions such as the proper amount of fat in a healing diet, the values of vitamin and mineral supplements, and the merits of drinking large quantities of raw fruit and vegetable juices. Many surveys find that raw juices are effective in combating disease. However, some physicians point out that the reason for positive test results is that the people drinking the juices tend to be more health conscious and to take better care of themselves in general. Others suggest that consuming the entire fruit or vegetable, rather than just the juice, is preferable. There are physicians who will advise a patient not to eat any animal products, while others claim that being vegetarian is dangerous to one's health. (It is certainly true that not all vegetarians are healthy.) I will not confuse you with all of these arguments, but

I will provide simple, practical suggestions about foods that favor the recovery process. The key elements of your diet should be fruits and vegetables, protein, and complex carbohydrates. First, however, let us examine the most readily accessible detoxifier in your disease-fighting repertory: water.

THE AMAZING POWER OF PURE WATER

Most physicians will tell you that drinking six to eight glasses of water a day is essential to support your body's power to cleanse, nourish, rejuvenate, and heal. An insufficient supply of water in your body creates disturbances at every level, from the proper functioning of the central nervous system to dehydration of organ tissue and thickening of the blood. The water in our kidneys permits us to remove deadly toxins that might otherwise be trapped in our systems. Depleted water levels in the brain result in mental confusion and headaches.

Next to the air we breathe, water is the most important thing we put into our bodies, but not all water is the same. Depending on the source of the water, it will have different properties you need to know about.

Most tap water in the United States is chlorinated, fluoridated, and chemically treated in various ways. The higher the fluoridation, the greater the likelihood that cell tissue will absorb toxic substances, such as lead from water pipes and aluminum from cookware. Moreover, despite government oversight, toxic chemicals and heavy metals used by industry and agriculture find their way into our groundwater, adding more pollutants to the water. For someone already suffering from a lowered immune system and its side effects, it is my belief that a clean source of water can enhance the recovery process. Distilled water, which is produced by reverse osmosis, filtering, or boiling, is perhaps the safest and most convenient choice because it is the purest of all water available on supermarket shelves.

LOW IN SATURATED FATS; HIGH IN FIBER

The foundation of your healthy eating plan will likely be a diet low in saturated fats and high in fiber. The primary components will be foods that provide your body with the essential nutrients it needs to function at optimal capacity. These nutrients include vitamins and minerals, protein, fats, and carbohydrates. Each plays an important role, so to ignore one at the expense of another is a mistake. Fruits and vegetables will be the major sources for vitamins, minerals, and fiber. They should be fresh and well-washed. Meat, poultry, and fish, the primary sources for protein, should be lean.

Trans-fatty acids—such as those found in margarine, vegetable shortening, partially hydrogenated oils, and certain types of vegetable oils such as coconut or palm—must be avoided, along with refined sugars. Incorporation of omega-3 fatty acids—such as those found in fish and in flax products—should be encouraged. Too many carbohydrates from processed foods slows down rather than speeds up the recovery process. The more whole grains and whole grain products you can introduce into your diet, the better. These recommendations are practical and sensible. They do not require you to become a food faddist or to give up familiar and popular foods. Most important, they will help your body heal itself.

These nutrition basics are all things we should know. It is important, however, to educate yourself further on how particular food groups can intervene in your personal recovery process. The foods you eat can nourish, and they can also heal.

Conversely, some foods do not contribute to healing at all or may have a negative effect. It is important to know the difference, or at the very least to educate yourself about what options are available. Challenge yourself to become an expert on what you put into your body.

LOTS OF FRUITS AND VEGETABLES

Perhaps the most potent and underutilized food group you will have in your diet are fruits and vegetables. They can not only accelerate body detoxification—remove toxin buildup—but they help to normalize body chemistry, the two most common problems related to disease and illness. Fruits and vegetables are effective because they contain phytochemicals and phytonutrients, which act in much the same way as the pharmaceuticals your physician may prescribe. Their advantages over pharmaceuticals are many. They are entirely natural; the body will more easily digest them; and as a general rule, they do not produce negative side effects. They can be rich in fiber, the indigestible residue in plants that is too complex chemically for our digestive system. Adequate fiber in the diet promotes digestive health and stimulates regular elimination.

Recent studies have confirmed what dieticians have long suspected. Eating even small amounts of fruits and vegetables at each meal will have beneficial effects and will boost the immune system. Studies have confirmed that the phytochemicals found in cruciferous vegetables, such as cabbage, broccoli, and Brussels sprouts, reduce the incidence of several forms of cancer. Tomatoes contain lycopene, an antioxidant that neutralizes roaming oxygen molecules known as free radicals, which are suspected of triggering a wide range of illnesses. The beta carotene found in red, yellow, and dark green vegetables bolsters the immune system and lowers serum cholesterol. Phytic

acid, an antioxidant found in sesame seeds, peanuts, and soy-
beans, enhances natural cell activity. Similar benefits can be
had from fruits. Citrus fruits in particular contain high levels of
beta carotene and vitamin C, which strengthen the immune
system, lower serum cholesterol, and protect against heart disease.

AVOID SATURATED FATS

A good general rule is to stay away from saturated fats. The difference between saturated and unsaturated fats lies in their molecular structure, and the scientific explanation of their
differences is more complex than is needed here. How do you
tell saturated from unsaturated fats? The easy way is to observe
them at room temperature. Saturated fatty acids, such as most
beef fats, are solid at room temperature. The greater the saturated fat content, the more heat will be required to melt them.
The lower their melting temperature, the greater the degree of
unsaturation. Fats from animals are the most highly saturated,
as are two vegetable fats—coconut and palm oils.

Saturated fats can damage many systems in the body. They
can clog the arteries and lead to heart and degenerative disease.
A high percentage of saturated fat in the diet stimulates the
liver to make LDL (the damaging form of cholesterol) in quantities greater than the body can remove from circulation. The
result is damage to the arterial walls, impairment of the cardiovascular system, and increased risk of premature death or disability from coronary heart disease. For people whose disease or
illness has already lowered their immune system or otherwise
weakened the body, the restriction of blood flow greatly de-
creases the body's ability to heal itself.

The least-saturated fats are found in corn, soy, sesame, sun-
flower, and safflower oils. Polyunsaturated vegetable oils, such

as those derived from sunflowers, sesame, and flax, should be used in salads and in the preparation of foods that do not have to be cooked. They contain good sources of the essential fatty acids necessary for proper cell-membrane function. Canola oil may be the best choice of all, because it is high in essential fatty acids and has half the amount of saturated fat found in other vegetables oils.

The middle range of fats consists primarily of vegetable oils that are composed of monounsaturated fatty acids, including olive, canola, peanut, and avocado oils. For cooking, olive oil should be the first choice because it is more resistant to oxidation and hydrogenation when heated than any other oil.

NOT ALL OILS ARE CREATED EQUAL

Pay close attention to the labels on the oil and oil products you buy. Many of the vegetable oils on market shelves contain synthetic preservatives and are heavily refined, bleached, or deodorized with chemical solvents. The more refined an oil is, the more processing stages it has passed through. Degumming may prevent oil from going rancid, but it also removes many nutrients, such as vitamin E. As a general rule, it is better to use oils that are mechanically pressed and the least processed. These oils generally have some sediment and taste of the raw vegetable from which they were derived. Unfortunately, these unrefined oils can easily become rancid. Purchase them in smaller bottles and store them in a dark cupboard or in the refrigerator.

You have many dietary options for making sure that you have enough protein in your diet. If you choose meat, fish, or poultry, you should be aware that there are saturated fats and potentially harmful toxins in all of these food groups. Think in terms of the food chain. Plants and lower-form organisms obtain their energy directly from the sun. Herbivores get their energy from eating the plants. Carnivores get it from eating the flesh of herbivores. The more stages through which the protein passes, the larger the doses of toxins that will be collected and then consumed. In most cases these toxins are stored in our fat cells.

RED MEATS ARE HIGH IN SATURATED FATS

Red meats and pork are high in saturated fats and are often polluted with toxins from the food and water that the livestock have been fed. Like processed or heated fruits, cooked red meats and pork form acid in the body, creating chemical compounds that can contribute to illness. This is above all a buyer-beware issue, and not just because of mad cow disease. Government labeling requirements on processed meats do not necessarily serve the consumer, and they allow meat-based products to contain many other animal parts in addition to meat. In most cases, the cattle and pigs have also been injected with growth-promoting hormones and slow-release antibiotics. Many packaged red meats and meat products have been preserved with nitrates, especially processed bacon and lunch meats. Not surprisingly, then, a hot dog is never your best choice for protein, because it may be comprised of many animal parts, including ground-up bones. Sodium, monosodium glutamate (MSG), and sodium nitrate are added to hot dogs in copious quantities. There are, however, healthful red meats you can buy. Purchase the ones with the least fat or marbling. Buy them at reputable grocery or health food stores, and buy them in their purest, most natural form.

One excellent form of protein is organically raised free-range chicken. However, commercially raised chicken can collect toxins from the food and water on which the chickens have been raised. The main advantage of chicken over red meat and pork is that the fat of the chicken, where most toxins collect, is external to muscle tissue and can be removed with the skin.

CHECK FISH FOR FRESHNESS

Fish is perhaps the best protein source, though many commercially marketed "farm raised" fish contain hormones similar to those found in beef, and even "wild" fish are exposed to many forms of contamination. Read the label and look carefully at the date on the package. Just because fish or meat looks fresh doesn't mean it is healthful. Many types of fish and meats have been treated with additives or coloring to give them the appearance of freshness. Labels may also indicate that certain fish, especially swordfish, marlin, and shark, along with shellfish, may contain elevated levels of mercury and other toxins. When buying salmon, you should always stay away from the farm-raised fish and go with the wild. The bottom-feeder fish are the least healthful. The fewer pollutants that you put in your body, the less difficult it will be for your system to direct its energies to healing.

Dairy products also bring protein into your diet. Here too, however, a person with a chronic or debilitating illness must be extremely careful in considering the potential benefits and the levels of environmental toxins, drugs, and hormones the products may contain. Just because a product has been labeled "natural" or "all natural" doesn't mean it offers complete protection. This is a serious USDA-labeling failure. Many cheeses, for example, can still be designated as natural even though they contain bleaches, coagulants, emulsifiers, moisture absorbents, mold inhibitors, and dyes.

BE AWARE OF LACTOSE ALLERGIES

When I was in high school my mother had a serious gastrointestinal problem. Even after she was hospitalized, she remained in intense pain and continued to lose weight rapidly, to the point where it appeared that she was melting away to nothing. We were led to believe that she was suffering from a grave and unidentifiable disease. Finally, after several weeks and after ruling out every serious potential cause of her symptoms, Dr. Joseph B. Kirsner at the University of Chicago diagnosed her problem as lactose intolerance. After treatment and after severely altering her diet, she eventually regained her health and the thirty pounds that she had lost. It was quite rare for lactose intolerance to be the source of such a complicated and life-threatening gastrointestinal problem. Dr. Kirsner's recognition of the dangerous potential of milk and milk products was quite a pioneering diagnosis at the time, and my entire family was grateful for his insight.

As we get older, lactose intolerance can develop unnoticed and cause a myriad of illnesses. Many people—young and old— have problems digesting lactose, the sugar in milk, and lactose intolerance may be worse if you have other food allergies, autoimmune disease, sinus trouble, bronchitis, asthma, eczema, or gastrointestinal problems. Another concern associated with dairy products, especially those that have been processed, is the tendency for these products to form mucus. If cleansing is what you are looking for—and anyone undergoing chemotherapy or taking high doses of medication fits into this category—dairy foods, in general, must be carefully evaluated. A person struggling to maintain a healing diet might look for alternatives such as almond milk, or tahini, a creamy ground sesame-seed butter.

Not all dairy has to be avoided. Studies have shown that

raw, unsalted butter—not margarine or shortening—is a whole, balanced food that is absorbed by the body better than its separate components. Yogurt, which is dairy in origin, is a good intestinal cleanser and boosts blood levels of gamma interferon. However, care should be taken in making your egg purchases. The difference between nutrition-rich eggs produced by free-range chickens and those that come from commercial egg factories is remarkable.

Refined sugar, or sucrose, is to be avoided because it has been stripped of its nutritional benefits. Refined sugars include raw, brown, yellow, and white sugars. The danger is well known to health organizations, yet the number of food products that contain refined sugars keeps increasing.

JUST SAY NO TO MOST SOFT DRINKS

Drinks to be avoided altogether are soft drinks, which offer sugar-laden empty calories that have no nutritional value. Virtually every nutrition expert lists the health problems inherent in these popular beverages. "Imagine dumping seven to nine teaspoons of sugar onto a bowl of cereal," writes Dr. Walter C. Willett, Professor of Medicine at the Harvard Medical School, in his book *Eat, Drink, and Be Healthy: The Harvard Medical School Guide to Healthy Eating*. "That's how much sugar is in a twelve-ounce can of Coca-Cola, Pepsi, or Orange Crush. . . ." The additional caffeine in many sodas turns them into diuretics, which cause the body to flush water, the great detoxifier and nutrient carrier, out of the system. This may be why many soda drinkers get headaches, notes Dr. Willett: the brain, which is 75 percent water, becomes dehydrated.

Are diet soft drinks any better? Because they contain artificial sweeteners, diet sodas do not provide the sugar overload that regular sodas do, but sugar substitutes such as saccharin

(Sweet'n Low) and aspartame (NutraSweet) may be problematic, especially for people with sensitivities to them. The research regarding artificial sweeteners is sometimes conflicting and seems to change frequently. To my knowledge, no studies have been conducted on the impact that artificial sweeteners have on people with lowered immune systems, but common sense should suggest that you stay away from them unless you are sure they won't affect your condition.

Even though the FDA has put its stamp of approval on these sugar substitutes, there are better beverage choices you can make. A far better choice than any soft drink is tea. Research has shown that green tea in particular has a long and impressive catalog of curative applications. It can lower cholesterol, may protect against cancer, and contains high levels of antioxidants, which remove free radicals from the body. In short, it helps to cleanse and boost the immune system.

VITAMIN AND MINERAL SUPPLEMENTS

If you eat a healthy and balanced diet, do you really need to take vitamins? The common argument that some health organizations and physicians use to disparage supplementation rests on the assumption that since obvious signs of vitamin and mineral deficiencies have been eliminated in our population at large, supplementation is unnecessary. That is true as far as it goes—deficiency diseases such as scurvy and beriberi have been eliminated in North America.

Not enough is known, however, about the less obvious deficiencies that give rise to disease and illness. This is a rapidly expanding field of research. Spina bifida, for example, is a crippling birth defect characterized by incomplete closure of the spinal column. It is also increasingly uncommon. Two decades ago no one knew that we could reduce the incidence of spina bifida by 70 percent just by giving folic acid supplements to women of childbearing age. Today, physicians risk being charged with malpractice if they don't recommend folic acid supplements to their female patients between the ages of eighteen and forty-five.

I am a strong supporter of supplementing a healthy diet with additional vitamins, herbs, and minerals. When I was first diagnosed with multiple sclerosis, I found that vitamins were my savior. At that time, there were no drugs or therapies to help me, so I turned to a combination of vitamins to improve my energy level and overall health. I have since added other supplements to balance and enhance my life. For example, vitamin C gives me enormous amounts of energy and supports my immune system to fight off various diseases. Evening primrose oil helps to balance my hormone levels. I can tell that my immune system is also supported. Calcium, of course, is good for everyone's bones and is especially important for women to combat osteoporosis. Vitamin D provides numerous general health benefits and is especially important in dealing with MS. I also take beta carotene and slo-magnesium. Finally, a relatively new supplement, CoQ10, is an amazing antioxidant that has been effective in keeping me healthy. These supplements can be powerful tools to ensure that the body is getting what it needs on a daily basis. To use supplements safely, consult your physician, carefully weigh your nutritional needs, and scrutinize the merits of each particular product.

STUDY THE NUTRITIONAL VALUES OF VARIOUS FOODS

In today's agribusiness, powerful chemicals are used to speed up a plant's natural growth cycle, and genetic engineering is used to improve the appearance and longevity of produce. Your impression of how fresh, green, or appealing a particular fruit or vegetable may look in the supermarket is not the best indication of its nutritional value. The leafy green vegetables and fresh tomatoes in a salad are only as nutritious as the soil and other environmental conditions in which they were grown. Do your homework. You may find that the most effective way to gain the nutrition you need is to supplement your diet with vitamins and minerals that can be purchased at pharmacies, supermarkets, and health food stores.

Perhaps the most important therapeutic ingredient in some supplements is chlorophyll—the pigment that plants use to carry out the process of photosynthesis. Chlorophyll is recommended for anemia fatigue, insomnia, exhaustion, nervous irritability, and skin ulcers and other skin disorders, and helps in coping with deep infections. A U.S. Army study revealed that a chlorophyll-rich diet doubled the life span of animals exposed to radiation—something that all of us undergoing X-rays might consider.

Finding alternative ways to enrich your diet is a gradual process. You do not have to do it all at once. The first and most important task is to learn what you can do to improve your nutrition, and then incorporate what you learn into your daily diet. Don't rush into anything you don't understand. Your eating habits have developed over many years and may be closely tied to family and cultural traditions. Trying to change such habits all at once is unrealistic and can be unpleasant as well. The changes need to be small and gradual. Keep accurate records, read labels, and pay attention to the results. Not everything you try will work for you. Give yourself a trial period of at least seven days with any new food or supplement. If you feel comfortable, add another innovation and allow a new pattern to evolve.

Most important: listen to your body. I think that you will notice quickly the positive benefits of healthy eating. A healing diet is both the least difficult and the most effective change you can make in your life immediately. Changing habits of a lifetime will require willpower and determination. Consider, however, that this is a relatively easy and rewarding step in taking charge of your life. Choose health with everything you put into your body. Eat right and live long!

Step Six Summary

1. Change to a healthy, healing diet.
2. Do not smoke, drink, or take drugs.
3. Research nutrition from authoritative sources.
4. Consult your doctor about all dietary changes.
5. Drink six to eight glasses of pure water every day.
6. Eat organically grown fruits and vegetables.
7. Do not eat saturated fats in meats and oils.
8. Eat energy-supporting protein in chicken, fish, eggs, grains, and beans.
9. Avoid refined sugar and artificial sweeteners.
10. Use vitamin and mineral supplements as needed.
11. Be an educated nutrition consumer and listen to your body.

STEP SEVEN

Let's Get Physical

No matter who you are, you have plenty of options in the area of physical health. There are many exercises you can do, regardless of the physical limitations caused by your condition. Virtually all of them will help reduce major obstacles that can interfere with recovery: fatigue, stress, anxiety, muscle pain, and lack of sleep. Following a healthy exercise program will improve circulation, pump needed oxygen into your bloodstream, stimulate production of healing hormones, reduce the risks of heart attack and cancer, build muscle tissue, reduce body fat, and improve strength and endurance. These are just a few of the more obvious benefits.

A less understood but equally important benefit is that exercise can be an important spiritual activity—a mechanism for uniting the mind, body, and spirit into a healing force. This mind/body connection can be as potent as a standard medical treatment plan. People of any faith can use exercise and a greater awareness of the connection between mind and body to pump up their immune systems and to direct blood flow to particular body organs or muscle groups that may need attention. Astonishingly, there are clinical tests that prove this connection.

To counter the effects of MS, it is important for me to encourage muscle memory, and I exercise religiously five to six days a week. With MS, the messages sent from your brain to various parts of your body can become muffled. Exercise is essential to maintain the effectiveness of the nerve-muscle connection to keep the body responding as it should, even when you are experiencing an attack. When I do not exercise for more than a few days, I begin to feel very fatigued and numbness sets in.

It is equally important to me to exercise in order to alleviate stress. When you have a life-threatening disease, it can encompass your whole being unless you consciously find relief. One of my best stress relievers is to work out on my elliptical trainer, then lift weights and do crunches or sit-ups. On other days, I do Pilates or play tennis. Whenever I feel that I can't handle an emotional situation, I get on my elliptical trainer and by the time I get off, thirty minutes to an hour later, easily 75 percent of my stress is gone—or is just a lot easier to deal with. Exercise enables me to make more logical decisions and the euphoria of a hard workout makes me feel good about myself. I absolutely love to snow ski and I do it whenever I get the chance. With MS, I feel much better in the cold weather. Gliding down a beautifully picturesque snowy mountain with the invigorating rush of wind in my face is my ideal version of exercise. Exercise encourages the feeling that I can do anything that I set my mind to do.

LISTEN TO YOUR BODY

The first step in putting together an exercise program is the same step I have described over and over in this book: *just listen to your body*. A brisk walk around the block each morning, coupled with stretching exercises and muscle toning, may be all that you want or require. That said, the ability to recognize how individual parts of your body are feeling and how they react to emotional and physical stress is a powerful skill that can bring rewards far beyond the release of tension. It is a primary way of exploring the intimate connection between mind and body, of opening pathways, which can speed the recovery process.

There are, in fact, entire spiritual philosophies and medical therapies whose main purpose is to open those healing pathways. Some, such as yoga and Zen, are many centuries old, while others, like bioenergetics and psychoneuroimmunology, are brand new. Each works very closely with physical and mental exercises geared specifically toward healing and the regeneration of the body. For someone who has not explored such philosophies or therapies, it is natural to be skeptical about their effectiveness. Meditation and exercise are clearly no substitute for penicillin. I urge you, however, to keep an open mind about the potential benefits of exploring the mind/body connection.

Dr. Herbert Benson, president of the Mind/Body Medical Institute in Boston and Associate Professor of Medicine at Harvard Medical School, reports that mind/body techniques can improve almost anyone's quality of life. Meditation, he says, may not cure cancer, but it can greatly help to relieve the side effects of chemotherapy. A leading managed-care organization, HIP USA, now covers several mind/body therapies, and Medicare will reimburse for certain relaxation techniques administered by psychologists. Many major hospitals now have dedicated mind/body clinics. Classes in yoga are available at YMCAs and health clubs across the country.

According to a government survey in 2002, nearly half of all Americans used some form of mind/body intervention. Even if you are unable to walk there are still many exercises you can do. From swimming to Pilates, from upper-body machines (UBMs) to hand weights—you can receive the same benefits as any anyone else, and gain strength in your body.

Hundreds of clinical studies have proved that the brain and the nervous system do not work in isolation from the rest of the body. Through chemicals called neurotransmitters, information is constantly being traded back and forth. Neurotransmitters travel along hundreds of miles of neuropathways in our bodies and provide messages to our organic systems and cells. They are responsible for sensations, feelings, memory, and emotions, just as they regulate blood flow, body temperature, and organ function. They work on a molecular level to bring about healing, or, conversely, illness and disease. The brain, which is the single most important controller of neurotransmitters, offers a virtual gateway to countless other tissues and organs.

THE MIND/BODY CONNECTION UNDER STRESS

For a person under stress from a chronic or debilitating illness, the mind/body connection most clearly manifests itself in muscle tension. Emotions such as anger can be linked to chronic tightness and discomfort in the neck and shoulders; pain and anxiety can focus on the muscles of the stomach and abdomen. The tightening of those muscles in the abdomen restricts digestion, which results in the reduced flow of nutrients into the bloodstream. Feelings of hurt and abandonment can be linked to tightening of the arteries, which carry blood from the heart to the rest of the body. Every contracted muscle blocks move-ment and hinders the recovery process.

In a remarkable clinical experiment, researchers demon-strated an actual relationship between the spiritual mind-set and physical illness in a group of patients diagnosed with med-ically incurable malignancies. The group participated in a six-week program of theory presentation and application of topics such as the interrelatedness of mind, body, and emotions, relax-ation, positive mental imagery, and physical exercise. The av-erage survival time of participants still living at the time data was being collected was 24.4 months, twice that of national norms for people with similar conditions. Even for those who had died by the end of the study, the average survival time was 20.2 months, still one and a half times longer than the national norm. These results demonstrated the value of the mind/body connection that practitioners of various Eastern traditions have known for centuries.

LEARN TO LISTEN

Learning to listen to your body is the first step in almost all the healing techniques that draw on the mind/body connection. This exercise is particularly well suited to people who have a debilitating illness or condition—it can be done in bed or seated in a chair. Listening may take only a few minutes. For the best results, you need to be comfortable and relaxed. A good preliminary way to release tension is to take a few deep breaths and try to push mental concerns into the background. Then close your eyes and focus your attention on what is going on around you. Listen carefully to everything around you. Become aware of the sounds of cars driving past on the road outside your house, birds chirping in the trees, or coffee perking in the kitchen. Make a mental list of everything you hear. Try to iso-

late one sound from another. Distinguish its particular characteristics. In five or six minutes you should be able to acquaint
yourself with these various sounds.

Then, shift your focus to your body and to the physical sensations you are feeling. Most likely, you will first become aware
of your breathing, your body temperature, and the weight of
your limbs at rest. If you concentrate, you may gradually become aware of other sensations as well: tensions in your neck,
back, or chest. Perhaps you will feel various cramps, mild elec-
trical sensations, or your stomach gurgling. Make a mental catalog of these sensations also. Once you have taken this process
as far as you think you can go, try to shuttle back and forth between the internal and external sensations. This skill requires
practice, but the more you do it, the more proficient you will
become, and the more solid a foundation you will be laying for
what comes next.

There are many similar exercises aimed at creating conscious
awareness of your body. One of the most popular is "body scan-
ning," in which, either naked or wearing comfortable, loose-
fitting clothes, you lie down on a rug on the floor or on a firm
bed. You then close your eyes and begin concentrating on your
toes. Many people find it helpful to picture their toes mentally
as they try to become aware of how their toes feel. Next, you
proceed mentally to scan your body. Work your way up slowly,
from your calves to your knees and up to your midsection, into
your arms, and finally your neck and head. The purpose of this
exercise is the same as the earlier exercise: to become aware of
and differentiate among all the various parts of the body and the
conditions they are in. However, this is a refinement, a subtle
step in awareness. In the process, you will discover that some
parts of your body feel more stress than others, and that energy
and heat are trapped in certain places. As you will probably
note, the body scan is also a meditation exercise.

Many people have turned these techniques into an important part of their daily medical therapy. They study anatomical charts, MRIs, and CAT scans to better familiarize themselves with where healing work needs to be done within the body. Then they use a combination of breathing exercises, meditation, and mental commands to direct healing forces to the problem areas. They do not just imagine the work they're doing, they write it down and draw diagrams, as I suggest you do. They systematically prepare lists of the areas they will work on, and then they work through them in their minds.

BREATHING FOR HEALING

Breathing exercises are perhaps the easiest of all the beginner-level exercises that can be used to promote the healing process. As in all exercises of this kind, begin by putting yourself in a comfortable position, either lying down or standing up. Your diaphragm should be relaxed and your breaths deep enough that your abdominal walls rise and fall with each breath. Place your hand on your abdomen. Inhale through your nose and exhale through your mouth. Notice whether your hand rises with your chest. Try to expand and completely fill your lungs when you inhale. Then, empty your lungs completely when you exhale, so that your hand truly rises and falls.

The process may be more difficult than you initially imagined. Many people with illnesses breathe shallowly, and they need to learn to breathe deeply. The goal is to hold your breath for five seconds, or to work incrementally toward that goal, and to balance your breathing so that the length of your inhale and that of your exhale are approximately the same. In theory, the more balanced your breathing, the more your body will seek to bring itself into balance. In these and other exercises, develop your technique slowly. Do not be upset if you cannot do the exercises right away. They require practice and time to master.

Meditation can be extremely effective when combined with breathing exercises. Following Buddhist tradition, "conscious" breathing is done with an attitude of good health and a love for yourself and all of life. Buddhist practitioners say prayers as they inhale and exhale. Particular prayers are tailored to the desired effect, whether it is relief from a type of pain or inflammation or a desire to strengthen the spirit. "If you can control the breath," a Zen master once said, "you control the mind. And controlling the mind is the gateway to the body." Breathing exercises are certainly not limited to Buddhists. With or without a religious orientation, meditation is a way to quiet the mind's chatter and to guide energy to blot out pain and to regenerate tissue.

THE MANY FLAVORS OF YOGA

Guided imagery exercises are also an introduction to more vigorous mind/body exercises, such as yoga, which focuses on developing control of the body through balancing body, mind, and spirit. There are hundreds, perhaps thousands, of yoga disciplines. No one style is inherently better or more effective than another; your choice may simply be a matter of personal preference or of finding a teacher whom you can relate to and a style that furthers your personal growth.

Hatha yoga, the most commonly practiced form, combines breathing exercises with a series of body postures designed for physical and mental benefits. These benefits can range from relaxation and stress reduction to better posture, better balance, increased lung capacity, and greater mobility. The act of controlled breathing—which increases oxygen flow to the brain and sets a rhythm within the body and mind—is coupled with poses that are held anywhere from ten seconds to a minute. At the core of all the poses is flexibility of the spine: forward-bending poses balance backward-bending poses; left twists balance right twists. The goal of yoga is to relax the muscles, but it also makes them elongated and strong. The result is good blood flow and dissipation of stress.

Because I have MS, if I participate in a yoga session or other form of exercise, I need to be certain that I am in a cool room with cold water available. If my body temperature rises to over one hundred degrees, I am likely to have an MS attack. For this reason, it is very important that when I exercise I constantly drink cold water to keep my body temperature down. This, however, is no excuse for not working out. I just need to choose my form of exercise carefully. Bikram yoga, which is done in a very warm room (to promote better muscle elasticity), is not for me. Yoga, however, is not my favorite form of exercise—I prefer something fast, with loud rock music to pump me up, and lots of cold water to cool me off.

People suffering from a chronic illness may wish to begin with a simple yoga style. Although stretching is healthy for everyone, the more aerobic the practice, the more competition there will be for oxygen in your system. The muscles that are engaged will consume the oxygen, while other parts of the body, such as the internal organs and the endocrine and immune systems, may suffer. Do your research. There are programs in many cities geared specifically for people with certain conditions, including fibromyalgia, chronic fatigue syndrome, cancer, Parkinson's, MS, and arthritis.

Regardless of whether you choose yoga or another mind/body form of physical therapy, lessons learned in studying them can be helpful when doing more traditional exercises, such as stretching, aerobics, and muscle toning. The less complicated and the more fun you can make your routine, the more likely you will stay with it. Also, the more you vary the exercises, the better you will work every muscle group in your body.

CONSISTENCY IS THE SECRET

With your exercise, as with your nutrition, the secret is consistency. Muscle deconditioning, a result of inactivity, leads to a myriad of problems and stresses the body. The heart, which is made of muscle tissue, can become deconditioned just like the muscles in your arms and legs. The heart becomes less efficient—it pumps less blood, less oxygen, and fewer essential nutrients to other parts of the body. Muscles that do not receive these essentials do not function properly and have more difficulty healing themselves. The more a muscle has become deconditioned, the less efficient it is in doing what it is supposed to do. That muscle requires more energy and oxygen to perform its activities, again robbing needed oxygen from such functions as building tissue.

Putting yourself on a proper exercise regime is not as difficult as it may first appear. There are plenty of simple exercises that can get you going, and the more you do, the easier and more effective they become. Running a marathon is not necessary. Just remember: every exercise helps. If you cannot go to the gym or jog around the block, you can simply walk or wheel yourself around the house. Lift a few weights. You can also use the edge of a chair or a bench to do incredible arm, leg, and abdominal exercises. There are even simple one-minute exercises that have proven effective.

REGULAR STRETCHING PROMOTES SLEEP

You may wish to begin your day with basic stretching. Starting out every morning with a few basic stretches will increase the flow of oxygen to your tissues, loosen your muscles, and help clear your system of the toxins and other waste that has collected over the night. Stretching before you exercise is very important to warm up your muscles and prevent injuries. Stretching in the evening before you go to bed helps promote muscle relaxation and a more sound and restful sleep.

Stretching exercises need not be vigorous or prolonged. The aim is not to produce cardiovascular strength, as in aerobics, but to increase muscle flexibility and joint mobility. These are always slow, sustained, and relaxing movements, which make them particularly good for someone who is bedridden or is in otherwise poor physical condition. They can be done in wheelchairs, sitting down, or flat on your back or side. They can also be done alone or with the assistance of caregivers.

The range of stretching exercises you will want to incorporate into your program may include arm circles, wrist circles, shoulder shrugs, calf stretches, knee raises, knee extensions, back stretches, and ankle circles. In general, you will want to hold a stretch position for thirty seconds. A full complement of stretches can be done in fifteen to thirty minutes.

A particularly good stretch for people recovering from illness is the back and hamstring stretch. This can be performed lying on the floor on your back. Keeping one leg straight, grasp the knee or thigh of your other leg with both hands and pull it toward you. After some practice you will be able to do this with both legs, touching your knees to your forehead.

The resources section at the back of this book lists many Web sites that illustrate these and other stretches. Most libraries also carry guides to stretching exercises. Once you have become comfortable with stretching, you will want to add a cardiovascular, or aerobic, exercise.

Doing aerobics increases your heart rate and blood flow and makes you breathe more rapidly and deeply than you would when performing daily or routine tasks. The benefits are numerous for people who have a chronic illness or debilitating disease. They include increased mobility—making it easier to get in and out of bed, the car, or a wheelchair—and greater stamina, which helps to fight fatigue. Any form of exercise is a great way to alleviate stress. Benefits are less noticeable in your metabolism, but still important are the improved blood-cholesterol levels and lower blood-sugar levels. No matter what you do, the exercises must be done at least three days a week for you to receive the most benefits. As with stretching, consult your physician to help you determine what is right for you.

BEGIN AEROBICS BY WALKING

A good way to start an aerobics program is to take a brisk walk for fifteen to twenty minutes a day. Research has shown that a daily walk, taken after your largest meal, is a sure way to increase circulation, energy, and strength, and to reduce stress. Many people also find this the most pleasant and relaxing of aerobic exercises. In walking, as in all aerobics, physicians recommend beginning at a moderate or low level of intensity. This means that you should be exercising at a level where your heart rate increases and you are breathing heavier than you would normally. If you cannot easily carry on a conversation while doing it or immediately afterward, slow down. The purpose of a moderate walk is to get your heart rate up, not to exhaust you. Always make sure that you are wearing the right shoes so that you may avoid any injury. There are many walking and running shoes to choose from. Just make sure not to buy the "fashion" athletic shoes for strenuous exercise.

In addition to a daily walk, dance is another great aerobic exercise. Legs and lungs both show rapid improvement, not to mention the fun you may have doing it. Any kind of dancing is a good workout, and the breathlessness you feel afterward is a sure sign of aerobic benefit.

Aqua aerobics, or just plain swimming, uses all parts of the body at once, so noticeable improvement comes quickly. It has many advantages over other forms of aerobics because your body is suspended in the water, which greatly reduces the stress on your limbs and joints. This may be the best exercise for many individuals with neuromuscular conditions, because it minimizes mechanical stress on the body. Most YMCAs, some health clubs, and many hospitals offer aqua aerobics programs.

Stair-climbing machines, rowing machines, and exercise bikes (or the real thing) also provide good aerobic exercise. There is a wide variety of these kinds of exercises to choose from to suit every lifestyle and range of physical conditions. Many people like to focus on one particular aerobic activity. However, you are free to change your workout routine to keep the process from becoming tedious.

AEROBICS CLASSES FOR THE ADVANCED

The most intensive aerobic exercises are those undertaken in group settings at gyms, dance studios, and health clubs. They can range from a fat-burning workout to a total-body routine— or Tae Bo–style classes. These workouts are invariably done to music, begin and end with stretches, and last about an hour. Such classes are widely available and held every day, at low prices. I urge everyone to look into this as part of their long-term exercise plan. If going to a gym or health club is not convenient, aerobic-exercise tapes and DVDs for home use are readily available. Some are tailored specifically for people with illnesses and special conditions, including those who are wheelchair bound.

OTHER EXERCISES

The last group of useful exercises is designed for muscle toning. Most toning exercises can be placed in one of two categories. Isometric exercises, which are a good way to begin, require the contraction of muscles against the body's own resistance. These exercises can be done without weights, by pressing your palms together at chest level. Another common form of isometric exercise is to push against a wall. Even though there is exertion by the muscles, there is no actual movement. Each exercise should be repeated five to ten times for six to eight seconds, three to five days a week. Isotonic exercises involve the contraction of muscles against resistance through a range of movement, such as weight lifting. Some good examples are crunches or sit-ups for abdominal muscles, partial squats for thigh muscles, and push-ups for arm and chest muscles. Isotonic exercises are especially good for increasing the size of the muscles or simply for toning.

NO MATTER WHICH EXERCISES YOU CHOOSE—from yoga to Pilates to dancing to tennis or sailing, there are important things always to keep in mind:

- Moderation is the rule. Stop exercising before you become exhausted.
- Consult your physician to develop an exercise routine.
- Choose a routine that is fun.
- Consider making positive affirmations a part of your routine.
- Exercise in a pleasant environment with adequate ventilation.

- Pace yourself. Plan out your program in advance.
- Incorporate flexibility into your routines.
- Set short-term, realistic goals.
- Drink plenty of water.
- Learn to listen to your body and pay attention to what it's telling you.
- Keep records for future reference.

Remember: Every exercise helps. Make them convenient and easy.

Step Seven Summary

1. Always listen to your body.
2. Begin with a mental "body scan."
3. Learn simple deep breathing.
4. Consider a form of yoga.
5. Maintain a consistent program of exercise.
6. Stretching can be good exercise.
7. Aerobics will strengthen your heart and lungs.

STEP EIGHT

Explore Alternative Therapies

MOST OF THE HEALTH CARE EXPERIENCES of my early life—with the important exception of one with my son Jason—were with traditional medicine as practiced by members of the American Medical Association. I had only a vague idea of what *homeopathic* or *holistic* meant. At that time, the concept of alternative medicine sounded like something very strange for earthy, new age, vegetarian, chanting types, not me.

However, when presented with the terrifying diagnosis of multiple sclerosis and faced with one conventional doctor's prognosis of "no hope, no cure, go to bed," and be a vegetable, I tried to learn everything I could that might help me.

Because there were no drugs on the market to stop the progression of MS at the time, I began to explore alternative and complementary medical treatments that are holistic and outside conventional medical practice. The alternative therapies I discovered rely on natural substances and methods to aid the healing process, are noninvasive, and cost a fraction of the price of more orthodox treatments. When I began my self-education in medicine, I learned how powerful and "normal" alternative therapy can be. Alternative medicine is not practiced by quacks or charlatans—a homeopathic physician goes to medical school for the same number of years as a traditional doctor, and in many cases, longer.

Most traditional doctors cannot believe how healthy I am and how my MS has remained under control. They can't wait to ask me which of the new MS drugs I am taking. When I tell them that I am not using any of the traditional medicines, they respond with raised eyebrows and immediately try to convince me that I am wrong to trust alternative therapies. They say that I must immediately go on one of the new MS drugs. I tell them that I trust my body. I listen to my body. Had those drugs been available when I was first diagnosed, I am sure that I would have tried one of them. They were not, so I learned to get better by a different route.

Right now, there are five drugs that have received FDA approval in the last eleven years for the treatment of MS. I am very happy that these drugs are available and I support the research that is bringing them and other therapies to MS patients. However, they do not work for everyone. For the people who respond well to them, they are lifesaving wonder drugs. If I were not feeling so healthy and testing so well, I might consider one of them. The fact is that when I have an MS attack, I go the homeopathic route. This is what is right for me. My body tells me so. It may not be right for you to emulate what I do. You must learn everything you can about your particular disease. Study every therapy and drug on the market. Then, listen to your body, and choose what is right for you. Often, this can be a trial-and-error process. Do not be disappointed if the first drug you try does not work for you.

Homeopathy has proven effective in treating my disease. Not everyone will want to follow this path, but I encourage you to explore your options. Just as you tailored your nutrition and exercise regimen to meet your individual needs, do the same with your medical treatment plan. Do not assume that the treatment your physician has recommended or your health care provider has selected is the right one or the only one for you. Sometimes, it is important to combine both schools of thought. You must know going into this that traditional doctors look down on homeopathic doctors and the reverse is also true.

WHERE I STAND ON ALTERNATIVE MEDICINE

Just to be perfectly clear, I want to state that I am not an advocate for either conventional medicine or alternative medicine. Both have worked for me. I continue to consult both types of doctors. My foundation supports research in conventional medicine because the scientific method seems the most promising way to explore new technologies that yield the secrets of the human body. There is much about the body that we do not know and do not understand. My instincts and my experience tell me that the best path for me embraces many models of health care. I listen to my body. You must do the same, and give your body what it tells you it needs. Be informed and be open-minded and willing to explore that which is not familiar to you.

A HOMEOPATH CURED MY SON OF EAR INFECTIONS

I was first introduced to alternative health care solutions when my youngest son was five years old. Right after moving from Denver to Los Angeles, Jason began to suffer from chronic ear

infections. From three years of preschool on through kinder-
garten, he missed several days of school each week because of
the constant pain in his ears, or because he was having an adverse gastrointestinal reaction to the antibiotics that had been
prescribed for the infections. Finally, after consulting at least
six doctors, someone suggested that Jason's ear problems might
be allergy related. Testing revealed that he was allergic to virtually everything. He was treated with allergy shots, which made
his skin break out in a painful rash. Nothing we did seemed to
help the whole problem. One part would improve, but the drug
would cause another symptom to emerge.

Eventually I heard about a homeopath, a doctor who practiced a medical philosophy that recognizes disease as being
caused by diet and other imbalances within the body. I was
skeptical, but I was also desperate to help my son, whose education was being adversely affected by the problem. I decided to
schedule an appointment. The doctor had a very unusual approach to an examination: He simply interviewed Jason and me
at length, took Jason's pulse, and then gave him something he
referred to as Jason's "constitution," along with some homeopathic supplements. This approach seemed almost ridiculous
compared to the extensive examinations and testing to which
the traditional doctors had subjected Jason. Astonishingly, he
was cured almost immediately. There were several tune-up visits, but these were directed toward strengthening his overall
health. Jason never had another ear infection after that first
visit. His skin rash cleared up and he stopped getting sick and
missing school. I was completely in awe of how this alternative
style of medical treatment worked. It made a real believer out
of me.

A few years after this experience I was diagnosed with MS.
My conventional doctors were intent on giving me intravenous
steroids—the only conventional-medicine option at the time

for treating MS attacks. I knew, though, that steroids can bring on diabetes in someone with a family history of diabetes, which I had. The last thing I needed in my life was two autoimmune diseases at once. I decided to find out more about alternative options, something I probably never would have done had I not had that experience with Jason.

STAY OPEN-MINDED ABOUT ALL THERAPIES

Today, despite my MS, I maintain my health in large part due to a combination of alternative therapies, and often I use traditional medicines for many other ailments that come along. I am not suggesting that you run out and find a homeopathic doctor to treat your MS or other chronic illness. What I am suggesting, however, is that much can be learned by being open-minded about alternative health methods and practices. In addition to homeopathy, the major alternative health care systems you should know about are naturopathy and osteopathy, which are significantly different from conventional medical practices. Learning about alternative therapies, such as chiropractic, acupuncture and acupressure, biofeedback, and hyperbaric oxygen therapy will further broaden your understanding. If conventional medical physicians had all the answers, these health care systems and therapies would be unnecessary.

You may explore these possibilities safely and sanely, without endangering your health. You are not going into uncharted waters. In studying alternative health care systems and therapies you may be surprised by their apparent simplicity and the ease with which you can avail yourself of their benefits. Many industrialized nations, including Canada, England, and Germany, have already made alternative health practices a significant part of their national health care systems. Today, at least a third of the population in the United States uses some form of complementary or alternative medicine, and conventional physicians are no longer as resistant to alternative practices as they once were. Increasing numbers of M.D.s are including holistic treatments and adopting some of the thinking and practices of natural medicine to offer their patients the best of both worlds. Some of our most prominent medical universities are integrating the teaching of homeopathy into their curricula, and they are spending big research dollars there, too.

ALTERNATIVE MEDICINES AT THE SUPERMARKET

Today on the shelves of pharmacies, supermarkets, and health food stores, you will find a large array of traditional herbs and many newly compounded alternative medicine supplements. Alongside the now-familiar bottles of multivitamins, you will find ginkgo biloba and turmeric, which have the potential to help mental functioning; echinacea, for boosting the immune system; St. John's wort, for fighting depression; glucosamine sulfate, helpful for arthritis; and CoQ10, a promising heart-helping remedy. Some of these products are brand new; others are part of a vast, unwritten lexicon of healing that dates back several millennia.

HOMEOPATHY IS THE NUMBER TWO MEDICINE SYSTEM WORLDWIDE

Homeopathy, the alternative health practice with which I am most familiar, is based on the premise that the body is a self-healing entity, and that symptoms are the expression of the body's attempts to restore its balance. Homeopathic remedies, which are low-cost and nontoxic, have been found to be particularly effective in treating chronic illnesses that fail to respond to conventional treatment and are a good method of self-care for minor conditions from colds and flu to bee stings and inflammation. These general-purpose remedies, available at most health food stores and many supermarkets, are what make homeopathy the second most widely used system of medicine in the world.

In Europe, homeopathy is commonplace; its practitioners are far more recognized and respected than they are here. In Germany, its birthplace, homeopathy is required training for all medical students. In France, all pharmacies are required to carry homeopathic remedies along with conventional drugs, and Oscillococcinum, a staple of many homeopathic remedies, is the best-selling cold and flu remedy in the country. I never embark on an airplane trip without taking Oscillococcinum, and I always take a dose when I am near anyone who is sick or when I feel the first signs of a cough or a cold. For me, it has been my biggest help in keeping healthy.

THE THREE ANTIDOTE PRINCIPLES OF HOMEOPATHY

Homeopathy is different from naturopathy in that homeopaths adhere to what are called the three antidote principles. These principles will at first seem confusing, or at the very least odd, and many practicing homeopaths themselves have difficulty explaining why they are effective. Believers in homeopathy argue that although a homeopath may not be able to explain the biology involved, the results speak for themselves. In addition, unlike the synthetic drugs that are dispensed by conventional physicians, homeopathic remedies do not have negative side effects. The reason why most homeopathic remedies have not been the subjects of clinical testing is that most cannot be patented, and therefore they have not been embraced by major pharmaceutical companies, which pay for such studies. That situation is rapidly changing, however, and NIH has invested more than $124 million to examine alternative medicines with clinical tests through a new branch called the National Center for Complementary and Alternative Medicine (NCCAM).

The Law of Similars

The first and perhaps most odd of the homeopathic antidote principles is the law of similars. This often repeated principle, in practical terms, means that the same substance that in large doses produces the symptoms of an illness or condition, in very minute doses can cure it. Homeopathic remedies hence contain a tiny amount of the active agent of what might cause an illness. If the symptoms of a cold, for example, are similar to poisoning by mercury, then an extremely tiny amount of mercury might be introduced in a remedy to cure the cold. *Nux vomica*, a homeopathic remedy, includes trace amounts of the substance that causes cramps and vomiting. If given to a patient in a very small dose, it helps relieve cramps and prevents nausea.

The Law of Infinitesimal Doses

The second antidote principle is the law of infinitesimal doses. In other words, the more a remedy is diluted, the greater its potency. Homeopaths will therefore use only a small fraction of a substance, compared to what a traditional M.D. would prescribe. "Infinitesimal" is meant quite literally—there might be one part medicine to a trillion parts of water in a homeopathic remedy.

Each Illness Is Specific to the Individual

The third antidote principle of homeopathy may be summed up as "each illness is specific to the individual." This means that what is right for one person will not necessarily be right for another. Thus, in order to properly diagnose a patient, a homeopath will have to examine all aspects of a patient's diet and lifestyle and the many environmental factors that influence his or her health. In the case of headaches, for example, homeopathy recognizes two hundred symptom patterns, and has corresponding remedies for each. An office consultation can become quite involved. After recording the patient's case history, the homeopath will analyze the whole picture. By comparing the symptoms to the known remedies, the homeopath will then seek to find the single remedy that best covers the patient's expressed symptoms.

∞

THE GROWING SUCCESS of homeopathy as an alternative or complementary health practice is fueled by several factors:

- Homeopathy is extremely effective for many conditions, and the results can be rapid, complete, and permanent.
- Homeopathy is quite safe. Even babies and pregnant women can use homeopathic remedies without the danger of side effects. (But you must always consult your homeopath and obstetrician.)
- Homeopathic remedies use all-natural substances and are not addictive.
- Homeopathic remedies work in harmony with a person's immune system.
- Homeopathy is holistic. It treats all the symptoms as one,

which in practical terms means that it addresses the cause, not the symptoms.

NATUROPATHY OFFERS A
VARIETY OF CHOICES

Another good alternative health discipline to consider is naturopathy, which many people believe combines the best of both conventional and alternative medicine. Naturopathy has a long track record for being effective in the treatment of chronic and degenerative diseases. Along with homeopathy, it is one of the fastest growing of all the alternative health practices. Thirteen states currently license naturopathic physicians, identified as N.D.s; naturopathic therapists, educators, and physicians practicing naturopathic techniques can be found in all fifty states. Although the experience and educational requirements are different depending on where training and certification has taken place, all licensed naturopathic physicians have attended a four-year graduate-level naturopathic medical school. In addition to the same standard medical training in the basic sciences as M.D.s get, they are required to study clinical nutrition, acupuncture, homeopathic medicine, and botanical medicine. They also must attend psychology counseling programs designed to help them encourage patients to make lifestyle changes.

JUDGE AN N.D. BY THE SAME
STANDARDS AS AN M.D.

N.D.s have offices and examination rooms as do M.D.s, and they practice many of the same time-honored methods of consultation, case history, physical examination, and laboratory analysis. Please be advised, however, that naturopathic practitioners are not M.D.s, and that naturopathy, like many other alternative health services, is not covered by Medicare or most insurance policies. In judging naturopathic physicians or any other alternative health practitioners, use the same guidelines as you would when choosing your general practitioner. The more education and training they have received, the better. Find out which schools they have attended, which state licensing tests and board certifications they have passed, and what additional training they have received. Also, understand that just because a physician is a naturopath, he or she is not necessarily knowledgeable about other alternative health therapies. However, in all likelihood you will find that there is a great deal of crossover training.

A licensed N.D. may also have credentials as an osteopath and/or as a homeopath, and may further specialize in another alternative therapy. In the best of all worlds, you will want an alternative practitioner who is also an M.D. They are not necessarily easy to locate, but there are resources, which I list in my bibliography, to help you find them. A leading naturopath in La Jolla, California, for example, is also an M.D., and is a board-certified homeopath. A leading pediatrician in Santa Fe, New Mexico, has credentials as a naturopath and is also an advocate of hyperbaric therapy. The homeopath I consult in Santa Monica, Dr. Michael Galitzer, is an M.D. and has studied a wide variety of other alternative therapies, including naturopathy.

AID THE BODY IN HEALING ITSELF

Naturopaths base their practices on the premise that disease and illness should be treated by stimulating the body's ability to heal itself. In this and other alternative health modalities, the body is believed to have considerable power to heal itself, and the role of the alternative health practitioner is to facilitate that process with the aid of natural, nontoxic therapies. The concept of these therapies is thought to be integral to the healing process because our bodies are genetically designed to be compatible with healing substances found in nature. According to naturopathic theory, to introduce foreign or synthetic agents into the process may create greater imbalance.

Naturopaths further believe that disease, illness, and their signs and symptoms are manifestations of the body's attempt to heal itself naturally. Fever, for example, is viewed as just one of the body's ways of dealing with an imbalance. If the cause of the imbalance is not removed, the cause of the inflammatory response will continue, or will manifest in a different condition. The patient is viewed and diagnosed as a whole. In other words, a naturopath doesn't treat one organ, one set of tissues, or one skin condition. The entire body must be treated because all living parts are intricately related.

Naturopathic remedies and treatments invariably include careful attention to all aspects of diet and lifestyle. Herbal and mineral supplements, as well as vitamins, are often included as tonics and nutritive agents to support and strengthen weakened systems. Dosages of the remedies are always rather low and are never meant to give you side effects, such as the problems that often arise with traditional antibiotics and other pharmaceuticals. Hydrotherapy, Chinese medicine, and massage are sometimes made part of the overall treatment, along with many standard health treatments. Radiation may be used for diagnosis, but not for treatment. Major surgery and synthetic drugs are excluded from naturopathy altogether.

For many diseases and conditions, including colitis, asthma, and chronic fatigue syndrome, naturopathic physicians can be primary and even curative. In acute cases such as trauma from a serious automobile accident, orthopedic problems requiring corrective surgery, or emergencies of childbirth leading to Cesarean section, naturopathic medicine is not recommended, although it can contribute to the healing process. Like many other alternative health practitioners, naturopathic physicians function within an integrated framework. They can and frequently do refer patients to an appropriate medical specialist, such as an oncologist or surgeon. Naturopathic therapies can easily be employed within that context to complement the treatments used by conventional medical doctors. The result is a team approach that provides the best overall treatment for your specific medical condition.

PLEASE NOTE that here and in other discussions of alternative health practices, there are certain downsides that need to be considered. Many homeopathic remedies require great care in their preparation and usage. They are not like over-the-counter drugs in which one preparation is recommended for everyone of a certain age group or body weight. Each remedy is different and has been tailored specifically for that individual. Moreover, the sheer range of homeopathic remedies and the ingredients that are required can sometimes be difficult to obtain. Before you begin taking any drug, vitamin, over-the-counter remedy, or nutritional supplement, consult your medical adviser.

OSTEOPATHY IS A BLEND OF CONVENTIONAL AND ALTERNATIVE PRACTICES

The other major alternative health system you should know about is osteopathy, the oldest complete system of health care to originate in America. Today there are nineteen osteopathic medical colleges in the United States, most of which are associ-

ated with major universities, and more than forty-four thousand licensed osteopaths, designated as D.O.s, who have the
same license and scope of practice as M.D.s.

The appeal of osteopathy rests in its blending of conventional medical and surgical training and obstetrical practices
with osteopathic manipulation treatments. The osteopathic
system is based on the belief that the body is capable of making
its own remedies against disease and other toxic conditions
when it is provided adequate nutrition and favorable environmental conditions, and when muscles and bones—known as
the musculoskeletal system—are in proper relationship or
alignment. Similar to naturopathy and homeopathy, osteopathy is considered alternative medicine because it takes into
consideration not only a patient's physical symptoms and medical history but his or her lifestyle, attitudes, and environment.

Dr. Leon Chaitow, a leading practitioner in London, England, explains what led him to become an osteopath: "If you
consider that the musculoskeletal system makes up the largest
body system, using far and away the greatest amount of energy,
and if you reflect on the fact that it is through the musculoskeletal system that you live your life, you will begin to appreciate osteopathic medicine's importance. . . . At its simplest,
we can say that, when the mechanical structure of the body is
normalized or improved, it will improve in function."

It is this emphasis on the muscles and skeletal structure that
distinguishes osteopathy. The guiding principle is that "structure governs function," which means that the unique shape
of a particular joint or an organ will define how it should
move or operate, and if it is unable to move or operate properly, it will not function at its best. This principle, of course,
makes common sense when applied to joints and bones, but it
is not so widely appreciated when extended to all organs and
tissue.

OSTEOPATHS ARE TRAINED to look for particular symptoms caused by mechanical problems within the body. They make careful evaluation in four particular areas:

Posture and gait: How a person holds his or her body while standing and sitting and during such activities as walking.

Motion: Testing evaluates all moving parts for restrictions. For example, a patient may be asked to complete various body movements such as bending, side bending, extension, or rotation for both specific and general areas of the body.

Symmetry: To notice one-sided use of any part of the body and the subsequent stress that results. Osteopaths also look for increased or decreased curve in the normal spinal pattern.

Examination of the soft issues: Using visual inspection and palpation to look for skin cancers, hardening of muscles, temperature changes, tenderness, reflex activity, and excessive fluid retention.

IN TREATING PATIENTS, osteopaths utilize various forms of physical manipulation that allow the body's inner self-healing mechanics to operate more efficiently. *Cranial manipulation*, which consists of very gentle and subtle cranial massage, is used to treat conditions such as headaches, stroke, and spinal cord injury. *Myofascial release* is another massage technique that releases tension from the fascia—the elastic, semifluid membrane that envelopes every muscle, bone, blood vessel, nerve, and organ—thereby improving muscle function and restoring balance to the musculoskeletal system. *Articulation*, a quick, directed, thrusting pressure, is used when motion is severely limited. *Gentle mobilization* is exactly as it sounds: moving a joint slowly through its range of motion and gradually increasing the motion to free the joint from restrictions. All of these techniques can aid in the recovery process, though special care needs to be taken for people suffering debilitating illness or chronic disease.

CHIROPRACTIC THERAPY

Many people who are unaware of osteopathy as a medical system have explored a complementary form of osteopathic treatment: chiropractic therapy. Chiropractic therapy requires many of the same skills and training, even though it is not a fully articulated philosophical medical system such as naturopathy, homeopathy, and osteopathy. Be aware, however, that although a chiropractor may possess skills and training that seem similar to those of a conventional physician, he or she is not usually a full-fledged M.D. Here, as elsewhere, study a practitioner's credentials. The chiropractor you will want must be board certified and should have attended a reputable medical school. The more schooling, the better.

As with traditional doctors, there is no federal certification board for chiropractors. However, the Federation of Chiropractic Licensing Board will provide information about certification in your state. They can be reached at 970-356-3500 or on the Internet at www.fclb.org. You can also find a list of state certification associations at www.acatoday.com/about/state_assoc.shtml. The largest professional organization of chiropractors is the American Chiropractic Association, headquartered in Arlington, Virginia. They can be reached at 800-986-4636 or online at www.acatoday.com.

Many of us already understand that a chiropractor uses physical manipulation of the spine and muscle tissue to relieve pain and return energy to the body. The word *chiropractic* comes from the Greek *Chiropraktikos*, meaning "effective treatment by hand." The central belief of a chiropractor is that proper alignment of the spinal column—the central neural pathway in the body—is essential for the body to operate efficiently and comfortably. Chiropractic falls under the banner of alternative health practices in much the same way as osteopathy does, by placing an emphasis on nutrition and exercise programs, lifestyle modifications, and the mind/body relationship. This combination of therapies, and the generally lower cost in obtaining them, has made chiropractic the most popular of all alternative health practices.

Make sure, however, that you are going to a licensed chiropractor by checking the sources I provided above. This is a field with numerous frauds who give reputable practitioners a bad name. I see a chiropractor fairly often. When I am stressed out, I suffer from terrible pain in my shoulders and back. In a forty-five-minute chiropractic session the practitioner puts my back into alignment, and I feel absolutely amazing. My stress level goes way down and I leave the session feeling great.

∞

MOST PEOPLE FIGHTING A DISEASE suffer the consequences of some form of misalignment. This can result in a host of complications, including, but not limited to, back pain, asthma, headaches, and even hearing problems. Pain has the tendency to cause us to favor one side of our bodies over the other, or to affect the way we walk or move about. People who are confined to wheelchairs or who are unable to get out of bed frequently find themselves in awkward and uncomfortable body positions.

Chiropractic therapy may be a solution, or one of the solutions. Chiropractic should be viewed as complementary to other treatments of disease and illness; unlike naturopathy and homeopathy, its benefits for the chronically ill are more directly related to overcoming some of the secondary problems related to their disease, rather than tackling the main cause itself.

ACUPUNCTURE AND ACUPRESSURE

Having explored chiropractic theory, the body/mind principles found in acupuncture and acupressure therapy will not seem as foreign as they might otherwise be. Both are alternative health therapies that have been practiced in China, Japan, and Korea for five thousand years or more, though it has been only in the last century that they have gained respect in Europe, the United States, and Canada. They are based on a central tenet of traditional Chinese medicine: The body must be in balance to function at its peak. Emotional and physical energy, known as "Qi" or "chi," flows through the body along specific bioelectrical and chemical pathways called meridians.

According to acupuncture experts, major meridians, or channels of energy, run through the body, and each meridian is named for the organ or function connected to its energy flow. The body is considered in perfect balance when chi energy is flowing smoothly. If chi energy is slowed down or blocked due to factors such as injury, poor diet, stress, or environment, then physical or emotional illness results. The pathways regulate and coordinate the body's well-being by distributing chi energy throughout it.

Acupuncture and acupressure are relatively painless, non-toxic therapies for reducing and restoring chi energy flow. Many people with chronic illness or debilitating disease have been helped, especially prior to surgery and immediately thereafter. These therapies are also said to be effective in helping to rid the body of toxins, which is a serious problem for people undergoing traditional medical treatments that rely on synthetic drugs. Typical sessions last about an hour; treatment programs frequently require one to two visits a week for one to three months.

ACUPUNCTURE RELEASES ENDORPHINS

Acupuncture is different from acupressure in that acupuncture uses extremely thin needles to stimulate meridian points, often in conjunction with electrodes, to direct and rechannel body energy. Pain reduction is one of the most frequently cited benefits. According to acupuncture experts, needles stimulate nerve cells to release endorphins, the body's natural pain-relief substances. They also may stimulate the release of other chemicals and hormones that normalize body processes, which presumably is why acupuncture offers other healing benefits. In China, practitioners use it to treat everything from immune disorders, such as chronic fatigue, to allergies, asthma, and arthritis.

Enthusiasts for acupuncture say that it is especially effective in treating rheumatoid arthritis. Often, acupuncture is used in combination with complementary treatments such as heat therapy, in which certain herbs, like Chinese wormwood, are burned near acupuncture points to radiate through the skin and influence the meridian below. "Cupping," another complementary practice, in which heated glass cups are placed over acupuncture points to draw blood to the area, is said to increase circulation. Acupressure uses the same principles and meridian points, but works through finger pressure, massage, and stroking rather than needles to effect stimulation.

BIOFEEDBACK: A MODERN ALTERNATIVE PRACTICE

In contrast to these ancient therapies is biofeedback, which is another popular alternative health practice. This therapeutic technique uses electronic devices to give auditory, verbal, and visual information back to the body about how it is working. However unusual it might seem, biofeedback, more than any other alternative health practice, has made the greatest progress in changing modern medical practice and research. It has accomplished this by showing that people can and do have the mental capacity to control their heart rate, body temperature, brain activity, and blood pressure. It has shown that people can deliberately choose to affect these functions. For the chronically ill, biofeedback has the added benefit of keeping us in charge of our treatment process: You can see and control the effect your mind has on bodily functions and make adjustments accordingly.

Biofeedback works by having a patient wired with sensors that are attached to a computer. This can be done at home or in a physician's office. By giving auditory or visual signals to his or her body, a patient can learn to control what are usually subconscious responses, such as circulation to the hands and feet, release of tension in the back, and heart rate. Biofeedback practitioners interpret change in the computer readings, which then help them to stabilize erratic and unhealthy biological functions.

Unlike some alternative therapies, biofeedback does not address or seek to directly control serious illness or disease. Rather, it is a therapy intended to relax and promote healing, and hence is practiced by all kinds of health professionals, including physicians, psychologists, social workers, and nurses. It has also been seen as a useful medical tool for controlling health problems such as asthma, chronic fatigue, epilepsy, drug addiction, and chronic pain.

THE EFFECTS OF BIOFEEDBACK are measured by:

- Monitoring skin temperature influenced by blood flow
- Monitoring galvanic skin response
- Observing muscle tension with an electromyogram (EMG)
- Tracking heart rate with an electrocardiogram
- Using an electroencephalogram (EEG) to monitor brain-wave activity

THERE ARE OTHER NEW THERAPIES you may want to research. *Enzyme therapy* has successfully been used to remedy digestive problems. *Magnetic field therapy* can be used in both diagnosing and treating physical and emotional disorders, and has been recognized to relieve symptoms and, in some cases, retard the cycle of new disease.

The best way to begin exploring these and other alternative therapies is to obtain a general reference book. *Alternative Medicine: The Definitive Guide,* by Burton Goldberg, is one of the most comprehensive. The advantage of this book over some of the others is that it also provides references for specific ailments and hundreds of self-help tips. *Complementary and Alternative Medicine: An Evidence-Based Approach,* edited by John W. Spencer and Joseph J. Jacobs is a 632-page reference work by two men who helped to create the Office of Alternative Medicine within the NIH. This is a conservative book based on up-to-date, government-sponsored clinical research. One of the newest (2004) guides is *The Natural Physician's Healing Therapies*, by Mark Stengler, N.D. This is primarily a detailed catalog of herbs, vitamins, and other alternative supplements described by an experienced naturopath, who provides a lengthy appendix of studies done on each substance.

Finally, another word of caution. Many physicians, however well meaning and well informed they may be about conventional medical practice, are not likely to embrace their patients' efforts to explore alternative therapies. My traditional doctors rarely agree with what I am doing, although they are quite impressed by my progress. They are honest in saying that they wished other MS patients were doing half as well as I am.

Step Eight Summary

1. Be open to all health care possibilities that may help you—conventional and alternative.
2. Research alternative medicine and alternative practitioners as thoroughly as you will research conventional medicine and conventional doctors.
3. Always tell your primary consulting physician, who will probably be a conventional M.D., about all of your health care decisions, including diet, exercise, pharmaceuticals, specialists' recommendations, and complementary or alternative therapies.
4. Ask for your doctor's views on any alternative therapy you are considering: the risks, benefits, side effects, and interactions with medications you are presently taking.
5. Speak with others who have tried the alternative treatment that you are considering; you can find them by asking your friends, or by contacting discussion groups affiliated with hospitals, or through the Internet.

6. As with everything you do in your journey back to health, keep detailed records. Record whom you consulted, which medicines you took or therapies you were given, and any changes you observed. Share this information with both your PCP and your alternative practitioner.

7. If your first experience does not bring results, be willing to explore further.

8. Listen to your body. It will be your best guide on the journey to health.

STEP NINE

Tame the Health Care Monster

MOST OF THE PHYSICIANS, nurses, and other practitioners on your medical team will be dedicated, competent professionals committed to helping you overcome your illness. The health care bureaucracy in which they work, however, is a creature of another kind. The paperwork, red tape, and bureaucracy in the health care industry can drive you to distraction, and distract you from your ultimate goal: getting the health care you need. You virtually need a master's degree in red-tape reduction before you can even begin to navigate the serpentine corridors leading from your general practitioner's office to see a specialist.

No one who has gone beyond receiving his or her initial diagnosis needs be told about the long lines in physicians' waiting rooms, the multitude of questions that go unanswered, and the test results that you never get to see for yourself or don't understand. The lack of coordination at all levels of the health care industry—and the mountains of paperwork that result—is truly a monster that needs to be wrestled to the ground.

Whether you are the poorest person, the richest person, or somewhere in between, you should be entitled to the right medicine or surgery you need for your particular diagnosis. We each have one life to live, and this is our most precious right. Your financial situation should not determine your God-given right to live. Ironically, both the very wealthy and the very poor can get inferior health care for different reasons. If you are poor and uninsured or underinsured, there can be a tendency to skip expensive tests or procedures that a hospital or doctor's office will simply have to absorb. Conversely, if you are wealthy, some health care people see you as an ATM machine. It is almost as though you have dollar signs tattooed on your forehead. Because you can pay and might make a donation, there is an opposite tendency: Heap it on! I have seen so many wealthy people be "over-cared for," over-tested and recommended to do surgeries and tests that are not completely necessary just because they can afford it. This is just as dangerous as not having the right tests ordered because you cannot afford it.

When you wake up and see the hospital's director of development standing at your hospital-room door with a bouquet of flowers and a big smile, you know you are in trouble.

Put a human face on that monster and then train it to do the heavy lifting for you. The process is easier than you think, but you must take the time to understand the rudiments of how the health care industry works, the medical terminology it uses, the complex medical billing codes, and hospital and physician billing practices. If you take a few commonsense precautionary measures, the beast lurking in those medical-facility corridors can actually become your friend.

HEALTH CARE MONSTER TAMING, 101

The advice in this chapter will probably seem more difficult and complicated than any I have given thus far. That is because the health care providers have made the intricacies of health care finance so complicated. Be patient. Get help. Go slowly. This step concerns both your physical health and your financial health. Here is an overview of the material you need to know:

- First, understand the specifics of your health coverage. It won't be easy, especially at first. Find a person who works with your insurance provider who is willing to explain those aspects that are not clear (often deliberately) in the fine print.
- Second, learn the language of the medical profession. There are words and phrases that will greatly assist in your communications with both your doctors and the health care financial professionals. If you have some command of the specialized lingo, you will be better attended and more respected.
- Third, meet with the billing administrator in your PCP's office. Before that meeting, study the basics of the diagnostic and reimbursement codes, so that you will have a foundation for discussion.
- Make an appointment with the administrator of the hospital where your PCP and specialists practice. After a discussion of the medical and administrative aspects of their services, ask to be introduced to someone in the accounting department with whom you may have a discussion similar to the one with your doctor's billing administrator.
- As you develop a relationship with your doctor, make him or her your partner, not your adversary, in dealing with the health care establishment. Your doctor can help you control costs on a visit-by-visit basis by making careful decisions about tests, procedures, medications, and specialists.
- Set up a separate system of bookkeeping for your medical costs, if necessary with the help of your accountant or

financial consultant. However you do it, keep specific records of names, dates, phone calls, and details. You will always need a paper trail.

- With the help of your accountant or financial adviser, prepare a monthly analysis of your personal health care costs. You need to know where the money is going on a regular basis.

- If you do not have insurance and need to have a surgery or procedure, often you can make a deal with the hospital by paying in advance to obtain a discount.

———

START BY UNDERSTANDING your health insurance coverage: the type of plan you have, which costs it covers, and which costs are excluded. Knowledge is power. Do not rely on the glossy booklets that plan members are provided with. It is the actual contract itself—the one with small print—that governs the plan. This is the document that you will need to interpret the mass of paperwork and billing statements on which the system operates.

To understand health insurance coverage is just as important for young people as it is for older people. When you graduate from high school or college is usually the first time that you must learn the importance of buying a good health-care policy. People in their teens and twenties are normally healthy and cannot envision the problems of a life-altering disease. However, health insurance is not understood when you are healthy. You are shopping for insurance to protect you in the worst-case scenario, a catastrophic illness or a life-altering disease. Do not try to save a few dollars by selecting a policy that provides less than full coverage. Buy your health insurance as though you are planning for a catastrophe, so that you are covered to the fullest you can afford.

FOUR KINDS OF HEALTH INSURANCE

Your health insurance probably falls into one of four categories: HMO, PPO, POS, or Medicare. The following section is a brief survey of these kinds of coverage.

HMOs (Health Care Maintenance Organizations)

These are plans in which you pick your primary care physician (PCP) from a list of approved doctors with whom your insurance company has contracted. The benefit to the consumer is that medical costs and preventive care services are available at a fairly low co-pay—the amount the patient pays to the approved health provider for each appointment. The downside of HMOs rests in the limited choice of physicians with whom your insurer has contracted to provide services.

In most cases HMO doctors are given a fixed amount of money every month for each of the patients assigned to them by the insurance carrier, regardless of whether they actually see that patient or not. This is one reason why many HMO patients feel that they get little time with their physicians: it costs the physician money to see you.

If you need to see a specialist, as virtually everyone with a chronic or debilitating disease will, a referral has to be sent from your participating PCP to the HMO for approval. The HMO will determine whether a specialist is justified in your case, and then approve or disapprove the request. This process may take as much as five to fourteen working days and will generate considerable paperwork. Here, as elsewhere, you need to do some research to determine if the specialist who has been selected by your PCP is the one who is right for you. Check on his or her credentials and experience prior to your PCP putting in a request to the HMO. The time saved may be substantial, for the process of changing specialists, once approval has been granted, can take months instead of days. Take the proactive approach by determining in advance whom you will want to see and why.

HMOs Require Approval for Hospital Visits. If you need to visit a hospital emergency room, you are generally assigned to a preselected ER/hospital that has contracted with your HMO. You may be required to call your insurance company before you are allowed to go to the ER. If you don't follow this procedure, or if you decide on the basis of convenience, you may have to pay a higher percentage of your medical bill. Plan ahead. Find out where the approved emergency room is located, note this in your journal, and make certain that your support team knows about it.

Don't Get Surprised at the Pharmacy. Your insurance company has already negotiated with drug companies and pharmacies to obtain discounts on certain drugs. If the medicine you are prescribed is not covered by your insurance, your physician has to fill out a "prior authorization" form to justify the use of this drug. The approval process may take several days. Again, you should take the proactive approach: Call your insurance company to find out if the medication you have been prescribed is on the approved HMO list, and if it is not, check on the status of your physician's authorization before making your purchase. Don't leave this responsibility to your doctor. He or she can't be expected to keep apprised of the never-ending changes in the rules and regulations of each of his patient's insurance plans, and each insurance company's drug formulary—the list of prescription drugs that your policy will cover—is constantly being revised.

Prior Authorization Is Key in HMOs. Prior authorization also applies to testing and treatments that your PCP and specialists recommend. Find out in advance what is covered and what is not. In most cases, your PCP or specialist will have to fill out a request form and have this approved in advance. There can sometimes be delays before a test or treatment is approved. You must wait for approval, or be willing to pay for the test or treatments yourself. In the event that approval is not given, you can appeal the decision and take your complaint to higher authorities. If such treatment is still denied and you have exhausted the appeals process, you may wish to bring in an attorney or consult a health advocacy group. Some treatments and clinical trials are also offered for free or at a reduced rates through teaching hospitals or medical clinics. There are always options if you look for them. The first source of information should be your physician, but ultimately it will be your responsibility to do your research.

HOSPITAL VISITS ARE TIGHTLY CONTROLLED by HMOs. Typically, you or your physician must notify your insurance company in advance before they will authorize coverage for surgery or treatment. Just as your physician has negotiated a set fee for treating you, so have the billing departments at the hospitals. This is why most plans designate which hospital and specialist you must use to receive coverage. This often results in efforts made to have your hospital stay as short as possible. The less time you spend in a bed, using up medical resources and the services of doctors, nurses, and others, the more money the hospital gets to keep when your insurance company makes payment. This can be quite difficult for the patient who really would benefit from more days with attentive nursing care after a surgery. Often, you don't have the strength to care for yourself and may need various types of medical assistance.

Controlling length-of-stay (LOS) is an important part of a

hospital administrator's job. In the event that you feel you are not ready to leave the hospital, you must file an appeal. Through the approval process, your physicians will have to assure the insurance company that your admission and continued presence in that hospital is medically necessary. Diagnostic testing may become a problem if your condition has not yet been identified, or if your diagnosis falls outside the scope of routine HMO procedures. You and your physician may have to put up a fight for such testing.

PPOs (Preferred Provider Organizations)

Typically, a policy holder in this system will have to pay a fixed out-of-pocket cost, or a deductible, for all care received, rated according to age and medical condition. After the deductible has been met, the insurer picks up all other costs related to services covered by the terms of the policy, with the exception of specifically designated co-pays. Policy holders are also given a list of participating physicians from whom they will receive heavily discounted services. Depending on the type of PPO, the insured person might have to pay for all or a portion of his or her visit. The advantage for physicians rests in their arrangement with the insurance company: they give the price discount in exchange for a higher volume of patients.

The advantage of a PPO for policy holders rests in the freedom to visit any health provider they choose, and the coverage they receive once their deductible has been met. The PPO member pays for the services that are rendered. The insurance company then reimburses the member for the cost of the treatment, less any co-payment percentage for an approved physician, from whom they will receive substantial savings. In some cases, the physician may submit the bill directly to the insurance company for payments. The insurer then pays the covered amount directly to the health care provider. Beyond the initial cost of the deductible, the disadvantage of PPOs rests in the greater amount of paperwork required to be filled out by the participant. It will be up to the policy holder to fill out the forms in order to be reimbursed for medical treatment.

POS (Point of Service Plans)

These plans combine the characteristics of both HMOs and PPOs. Similar to an HMO, you pay no deductible and usually only a minimal co-payment when you use a health care provider who is under contract with your insurance company. Also as in an HMO, you must choose a PCP who is responsible for all referrals within the POS network. If you choose to go outside the network for health care, POS coverage functions as does a PPO. The advantage of POS plans is that you can easily mix the types of care you receive. It encourages a policy holder to use network providers but does not require them to do so. Often, a person can add a POS plan onto an existing HMO or PPO. This can be a very good idea in the event that you need specialized surgery, such as a kidney transplant. Having a POS option on your coverage will allow you to go shopping for the best treatment at the best hospital, rather than accept one that has been designated for you.

Medicare

This insurance, which is federally funded, is for senior citizens. Everyone over sixty-five is eligible. You can choose a regular Medicare plan or enroll in an HMO that has a contract with Medicare to take care of you in their system. This has generally the same rules as any other HMO, but the "Medi-Gap" insurers tend to pay for drugs and preventive services, which regular Medicare generally does not. Medicaid, another federally funded insurance, is available to the poor or indigent. The federal government pays a certain amount to each state to run its own program. Both of these services have become so complicated that there are entire books to explain the details of their systems.

The reimbursement rates to doctors who accept Medicare are shrinking every year. Because so many physicians have opted out of the program, the offices of those doctors who still accept it as payment in full are generally crowded, and the services they offer are limited. For the doctors involved, reimbursement is not the only issue. Many physicians will not accept Medicare or Medicaid because the paperwork is many times greater than that required for HMOs and PPOs. The rules and instructions for Medicare and Medicaid alone run some 130,000 pages—three times the size of the IRS tax code. In addition, some thirty federal health-care regulatory agencies have their own paperwork requirements, as do state and local agencies and accreditation authorities.

Having some form of insurance, no matter how limited, is better than having none. There are, however, several steps you should take if your medical coverage has lapsed and you don't qualify for government assistance. Inform the physician or other medical practitioner you want to see that you do not have insurance. Often they will accept a lower rate for their services or offer discounts if you pay in cash. They may also be willing to charge you the rate that they would bill an insurance carrier if you had one. The same is true for hospitals. Many teaching hospitals also have programs that can help underwrite health care costs and treatment programs.

Some wonderful hospitals, like St. Jude Children's Research Hospital which was founded by Danny Thomas and is now run by his daughter Marlo Thomas, exist where no child will ever be turned away because they cannot pay. They don't expect you to. They truly want every child to get better.

SPEAK THE SPECIALIZED LANGUAGE
OF HEALTH CARE

Learning what your policy says and does not say will require that you understand the medical jargon that is used to describe procedures and protocols. The extra effort it takes to become conversant in this language will be time extremely well spent. It will be easier for you to make sense of the paperwork and bills that result from your treatment, and you can more easily address issues that may arise in the arbitration process. More important, mastery of the language of health insurance will permit you to communicate clearly your desires and needs in ways that your physician, health care team, and insurance company can understand. The ability to speak the language of health care is a critical tool you will need to request the help you want when you want it.

The best way to begin the process is to create a glossary of terms, conditions, procedures, and protocols. The Internet is a good reference source, along with your insurance company's brochures and some of the books suggested in the Recommended Reading section in the back of the book. Start your own list of important terms and code words that are directly relevant to your condition.

∞

HERE ARE SOME BASIC MEDICAL TERMS and acronyms:

Allowable costs: the expense of services covered.
Ambulatory benefits: reimbursement paid for medical services while you are not a patient in a hospital or other medical institution. These can include services provided at your doctor's office and other outpatient facilities and emergency rooms.

Assignment of benefits: this occurs when your insurance company sends payment directly to the person or facility that provides medical services to you.

Basic hospital expense insurance: this pays for room, meals, and some expenses for a certain number of days when you are admitted into a hospital.

Benefit levels: the most reimbursement you can get for a particular medical service under your policy.

Capitation: a structured system that pays physicians or hospitals a fixed dollar amount for each person in their roster of patients—whether that person uses the service or not.

Closed access: restrictions that indicate you must work through your PCP and be referred by him or her to any specialist.

COB: the acronym for Coordination of Benefits. Insurance providers figure out who pays for what if you are covered by more than one policy.

COBRA: the acronym for Consolidated Omnibus Budget Reconciliation Act, federal legislation that makes it mandatory for employers to keep their former employees on their group policies for a certain length of time.

Co-pay: the out-of-pocket amount you will pay for each type of service received when your insurance provider pays for the rest.

CPT: the acronym for Current Procedural Terminology. These are the codes used by the health care system on insurance forms and medical records to pinpoint the service or procedure for which they are billing.

DAW: the acronym for "dispense as written," regarding prescriptions for a generic or nongeneric drug or medication.

DRG: the acronym for Diagnosis Related Groups. This is a classification system used to determine the reimbursement level for inpatient services.

Drug formulary: the list of prescription drugs that your policy will cover.

EOB: the acronym for Explanation of Benefits from a health care insurer.

EPSDT: the acronym for Early and Periodic Screening, Diagnostic, and Treatment Services, for preventive health care for patients under the age of twenty-one.

Grievance procedure: the process your insurance company uses to handle complaints.

HFCA: the acronym for Health Care Financing Administration, the federal agency that governs Medicaid and Medicare.

Hospital indemnity insurance: the costs incurred during a hospital stay paid at a predetermined amount, regardless of how much your actual bill may be.

ICD: the acronym for International Classification of Diseases, the coding system used to identify your diagnosis on insurance forms and medical records.

IPA: the acronym for Individual Practice Association, a type of managed care plan where the insurance company makes a contract with a particular physician or a group of physicians to provide care for their plan members.

Legend drug: another term for a prescription drug.

Maximum out-of-pocket costs: the highest amount you will have to pay for medical services.

Open access: a type of insurance plan that lets you see other network doctors without going through your primary doctor first to get a referral. Also known as an Open Panel.

Out-of-network: health care providers who are not included on your insurance company's list of participating providers.

Portability: a provision that permits you to change from one insurance plan to another without being subjected to exclusions that might otherwise be used to deny coverage.

Preadmission authorization: permission from the insurance company before you can be admitted to the hospital.

Relative value scale (RVS): a complex system used to determine how much the insurance company will pay to a health care provider for his or her medical services.

Respite care: this is care provided to a person who requires a high degree of supervision and/or medical care, often used in connection with regular family-member caregivers.

Rider: additional language attached to your insurance plan contract that changes something written in the contract.

Third-party payer: this commonly means your insurance company, as opposed to the patient or employer.

Usual, customary, and reasonable fee (UCR): the most common charge for a particular medical service in a given geographic area.

Urgent care: the term used when medical care is needed right away but is not a life-threatening emergency.

MASTERING THESE TERMS and others will make it considerably easier for you to address insurance problems as they arise and more easily navigate the medical system at large. The insurance representatives, doctors, and the many other people in the medical community are not necessarily your adversaries. It is the system in which they function that has become a monster that must be tamed. If you treat the people you come into contact with on a friendly basis, find the people with whom you are most compatible, and speak their language, everything will go much smoother. The more knowledgeable about your condition you are, and the greater your understanding of the language and terminology they use, the more they will be inclined to help you through the process. They will quickly see that you speak their language and should respond accordingly.

RULES FOR MEETINGS WITH HEALTH CARE PROFESSIONALS

- Identify in advance the people who are "gatekeepers" in charge of your health care policy and what function they perform. Keep their telephone numbers accessible, and share this information with your designated health care advocate.
- Do not lose your temper no matter how frustrated you feel.
- Have your insurance policy account number, ID, and paperwork with you before making phone calls and when visiting a physician or a hospital.
- Keep a detailed list of your doctors, their phone numbers, and their addresses in your filing system.
- Keep a detailed list of dates of consultations and which services were provided in your filing system.
- Keep a record, including time and date, of all telephone calls.
- If any kind of promise or approval is made to you about your coverage, ask that it be put in writing. Always ask for the name of the person you are speaking with and be certain to make a careful record of the name, time, date, and substance of the conversation.
- Take a proactive approach by following up any conversations with letters stating your position, and thanking people when they have been helpful.
- If you are turned down for coverage, or have difficulties dealing with your insurance provider, always request that their decision be put in writing. This will force them to

provide you with a written rationale for their denial, which you then may choose to appeal.

• Many times you will be charged for items that should be covered by insurance. The expensive but excellent insurance policy that I had for many years began to handle my bills differently. In order to be properly reimbursed, I just kept sending the bills back, and eventually they were paid. Clearly, I should not have had to send everything back. However, if I had not paid careful attention, I would have paid for many improperly billed items. Fed up, I recently switched to another plan, which covers much more at less expense.

YOUR DOCTOR'S BILLING ADMINISTRATOR

As you may have guessed from the preceding section, your doctor may have different motivations regarding your treatment depending on the health insurance you carry. No one understands this better than his or her billing administrator. You can certainly express your understanding of the administrator's needs, but do not fail to point out his or her responsibility to meet your needs. Both points of view have to work together within the parameters of the system. Generally, you will find billing administrators rather matter-of-fact about the way the system works. However, they can be informative about how to deal with various aspects of health care billing. If you show some interest in and some knowledge of their area, they will usually be forthcoming with sometimes surprising shortcuts and tricks to keep the health care monster calm. Above all, show a little kindness and patience— these are people who get yelled at on a daily if not an hourly basis.

CODESPEAK: THE KEY TO UNDERSTANDING MEDICAL BILLING

One of the key elements of the billing administrator's job is the coding of diagnoses and reimbursements. Health care insurers usually have established policies about which codes they will reimburse and which ones they determine are not allowable. This is one of the key pieces of information you need to find out. The International Classification of Diseases (ICD) was instituted in 1900; today it is maintained by the World Health Organization and is updated every ten years. (It is some indication of how completely the medical profession is being buried in bureaucratic paperwork that most American health care organizations are still using the 9th Revision codes instead of the 10th Revision codes, which were updated in 1999.) Current Procedural Terminology (CPT) codes were instituted in 1963 by the AMA and are updated monthly. Recently, codes for alternative and complementary medicine, known as ABC codes, have been added. Further information on these codes may be found at www.alternativelink.com/ali/home.

Each diagnosis is given an ICD-9 code, and each procedure or treatment is assigned a CPT code number by a medical office worker. For example, an office visit might be assigned any of hundreds of codes depending on how the visit was viewed. If it was simply a preventive checkup with your doctor, the office visit might be assigned a code that is not allowable under your coverage. On the other hand, if you request an appointment because of a cough or a stomach discomfort, these visits might be assigned codes indicating symptoms of medical problems that would be reimbursable. It all depends on how you, the doctor, and the billing administrator view it. In the best of possible outcomes, the right code will produce a win-win solution for both patient and doctor.

KNOW YOUR ICD-9 CODE

Sadly enough, once you are assigned an ICD-9 code by your health care provider, it is virtually impossible to have the code changed. Even if a diagnosis is determined to have been incorrect, you may be labeled with a code according to the incorrect diagnosis that limits your access to procedures and medications. You, your doctor, and your doctor's billing administrator must work together to assign the correct code to your health care.

Needless to say, your health care provider is not anxious for you to understand these codes. In many cases, the ICD-9 code that you have been assigned may determine (i.e., limit) the procedures and medications that are allowable for your doctor to prescribe. Numerous CPT codes could be virtually interchangeable for the same treatment, according to interpretation. Some are allowable and some are not. You cannot expect to master this system by yourself. Code billing is a burgeoning medical-business subspecialty taught in schools; those who have mastered it are well paid. Should you or a friend have the time and the inclination, there are numerous books and Web sites that deal with this coding system labyrinth. However, even if your understanding is limited to how the coding system functions, you will be able to work more comfortably with billing professionals in doctors' offices and hospitals.

MEET THE HOSPITAL ACCOUNTING OFFICE

All of us would prefer to be healthy and stay out of hospitals. However, once you have been diagnosed with a chronic or life-altering disease, you must face the possibility that you will need the services of a hospital at some point. There are books on how to deal with hospitals as a patient, but to my knowledge, there are no current books on how to deal with hospitals as a paying customer. (One of the best short reports is "Decoding Your Hospital Bills," at www.consumerreports.org.) If your diagnosis leads you to assume that a hospital stay may be likely, get to know how the hospital accounting office operates well before you are admitted. Be a knowledgeable financial consumer as well as a knowledgeable health care consumer.

As always, be proactive. First, ask your doctor and your doctor's staff about the questions that might be appropriate at a preliminary meeting with a hospital administrator. Ask the staff to recommend by name a particular individual at the hospital with whom you should speak. Second, as usual, do your homework: Find out which medical procedures may be necessary for you in the hospital. Find out the parameters of your health care provider's insurance for these procedures. Talk with friends who have had experiences with this particular hospital and might be willing to show you bills for their hospital visits. This information could be especially useful if you know anyone with your diagnosis who had hospital visits.

∞

SOME BASIC QUESTIONS TO ASK a hospital administrator or financial officer:

- How is billing usually handled for my health care insurer? How soon after my hospital stay are the billings available? Can I be provided with a copy (usually at a modest cost)?
- Are there specific daily charges for "basic hospital expense" that can be explained in advance? Does my insurer cover this cost? Are there other "standard" costs, such as operating-room time, that can be explained in advance?
- Does the hospital allow you to bring your own prescrip-

tions from home? Can items such as boxes of tissues and gowns be privately provided to avoid hospital costs?

- If you choose to have a private nurse in the room with you at all times, can a properly certified nurse perform some of the functions normally done by hospital personnel, such as drawing blood or handling IVs?
- Is there a hospital ombudsman or advocate who can assist you in understanding billings? (You will want to have your own financial people audit the billings, but hospital personnel can be helpful in explaining elements that may be confusing.)
- Might the hospital have any specific suggestions as to how to control the costs of a hospital visit?
- Just know that it's the same as when you stay in a luxury hotel and you eat food from the minibar or make long distance calls or fax or have a spa treatment—your hotel bill can double. Every little thing you ask for in a hospital comes with a high price tag, down to the Kleenex.

DURING YOUR FIRST VISIT with a hospital administrator or financial officer, remember that in addition to obtaining information, you are establishing a relationship with a potential ally for the future. Ask for business cards, write down telephone numbers, assistants' names, and other contact information. Simply the fact that you have made the effort to see them before a hospital visit will be impressive to them. If you are pleasant, knowledgeable, and reasonable with your questions, you will win important friends.

If the day comes when you and your medical team decide that you need to have a hospital visit for a procedure or treatment, contact the people you have spoken with and let them

know that you will be in the hospital. It may be beneficial to
your visit in many ways.

A WORD ABOUT
PRESCRIPTION DRUGS

I am well aware that pharmaceuticals is one of the most con-
tentious areas in the health care business. I am also aware that
some pharmaceutical companies have been guilty of gouging
the American consumer. (By the way, if you suspect price gouging, you might compare the prices charged at your local pharmacy with those charged at other locations. You may be in for a
surprise.) An excellent resource to check the price comparisons
on more than one thousand of the most common drugs is
www.pharmacychecker.com. This site also has ratings and profiles for fifty mail order and online pharmacies in Canada and
the United States.

However, I believe that it also needs to be recognized that
American drug companies are doing the research and providing the drugs that are bringing better health to the entire world.
Most drugs are developed in the United States and there is a legitimate reason for the high cost of many of these drugs: It costs
at least $100 million (and sometimes much more) to bring a
drug through research, clinical studies, and FDA approvals.
Nine out of ten drugs do not make it to market because of medical safety issues. Thus, these companies are left to support all of
the development costs from the drugs they can bring to market.
Collectively, American drug companies spend more on research than NIH spends. If companies were not allowed to
charge substantial amounts of money for these new drugs, they
would be out of business. In their continuing search for miracle
drugs to cure devastating illnesses, these companies are creating a healthier next generation.

After as much as ten years in the approval process and another seven years before the patent expires, drug patents are available in the public domain. What have commonly become known as generic versions of patented drugs can be produced by other companies. What is not generally known is that some of these "generic" drugs, which are much cheaper, are not exactly the same as the patented versions. If your doctor prescribes a generic and it does not seem to be doing what it should do, go back and request a prescription for the original patented medicine.

Despite the depiction of drug companies as "bad guys" by politicians and the media, they are amazingly generous in a little-known way. If you have a chronic disease and need expensive medicines that you cannot afford through your health care insurance, Medicare, or any other way, write to the company that manufactures the drug you need. Explain your financial circumstances and the prescription drugs that you need. In many cases, companies have quietly provided the needed drugs to impoverished people for their lifetimes.

Another lesser-known way to obtain expensive medicines—including some that are cutting-edge and unavailable to most of the medical profession—is to participate in clinical trials. Your doctor or specialist will be a good guide to the clinical trials of promising medicines in your area. (If you are willing to travel to participate in trials, you may receive compensation for your efforts.) Although pharmaceutical companies each run clinical trials under their own rules, they are all regulated by the federal government. One of the best sources of information about all clinical trials conducted in the United States is the National Institutes of Health Web site: www.cc.nih.gov.

A few thoughts about clinical trials: First, many of these tests require that you have not been treated with other drugs or procedures before being accepted into the trial. Second, many of them are "double-blind" trials, which means that you will have a 50 percent chance of actually getting the new drug being tested; neither you nor your doctor will be told. The other 50 percent of the people in the test may receive an already FDA-approved drug against which the new one is being tested, or a placebo, which is an inert substance with no therapeutic value at all. Third, there is a wonderful "up" side to participation in such trials: If the drug proves effective in dealing with your disease and you are not able to pay for it, the pharmaceutical company is obligated to provide you with this medicine, free of charge, for your lifetime. There are many issues to be considered before participating in a clinical trial, and the NIH Clinical Center has excellent information regarding every aspect of clinical trials that you should read.

MAKE YOUR DOCTOR A PARTNER IN TAMING THE MONSTER

The best approach to use with your doctor in matters concerning money is to be friendly, but firm. Always ask your physician if there are other treatment options available for you other than those your insurance company recommends. If you are denied coverage for treatment you think you need, or are told that no other treatment options exist, have your physician state his or her position in writing. If you need a referral, procedure, or hospitalization, and have trouble getting approval, ask your physician and his or her staff if they have any suggestions on how the authorization process might be streamlined or what you can do to gain approval. In many instances, there are key phrases that you or your physician may need to use, such as "medical necessity," "bad faith refusal," "irreparable damage," and "not within the acceptable standards of care," which will speed the approval process along. Always make certain that the authorization to see a specialist has been approved prior to your appointment.

Knowledge of the financial relationships your insurer has with your physician will sometimes be helpful in ferreting out the roots of certain problems that may arise. Not surprisingly, a physician who is paid each time you visit will be more inclined to see you more often. A physician who is paid regardless of whether or not you come in will likely desire not to see you as often. Short of changing your health insurance policy, there is little you can do about this. However, there are tips and techniques you can use to make the most of your visits.

In many cases, a physician allocates about fifteen minutes for each established patient. New patients are usually scheduled for longer appointments. Not all of this time, however, is necessarily spent with you. A portion of your physician's time will be spent filling out paperwork and forms and reading over your patient history. Mindful of the limited time you will have with your physician, you will want to decide in advance what you want to accomplish during your visit. You must be clear and precise in your explanation of what is troubling you.

MAKE EVERY APPOINTMENT WITH YOUR DOCTOR REALLY COUNT

Prepare for your visit with your doctor as best you can. Think about what is most important to you, and organize your questions in advance. Write them down in order of what is most important to you first, so that you do not become sidetracked. Check off the questions on this list as you obtain the answers. Have your notes and insurance papers with you, along with copies of test results or recent X-rays. Bring a list of your medications, vitamins, and other nutritional supplements with you—and correct dosages for each. Be as thorough as possible.

Sometimes it is easy to forget a drug or a vitamin. However, that omission could be vitally important. Your doctor needs to know everything you are putting into your body.

When you finally get this precious time with your doctor, don't be vague or ask broad, open-ended questions. Be direct and go down your list of important questions. A doctor has only so much time to spend with you. Don't waste time talking about issues that do not directly relate to the purpose of your visit. Don't talk about the weather, the news, or how much you like your doctor's new tie or haircut.

Everyone hates waiting at the doctor's office, especially when the wait extends long past the appointed hour and you want to get on with your day. Sometimes doctors must deal with emergencies that take precedence over regular office visits—if it was *your* emergency, you'd surely want your doctor to put your treatment ahead of the regular appointments in the waiting room. Depending on the type of doctor and the number of emergency patients he or she has to treat, your appointments could be delayed or even canceled at the last minute. Very often an obstetrician/gynecologist will be called to deliver a baby. A cardiologist can run late because of emergency surgeries or scheduled surgeries that have complications. Sometimes, however, emergencies have nothing to do with it. Any number of doctors' offices will regularly double-book patient appointments because they believe that their patients will cancel or not arrive on time. Although it's true that your doctor's time is valuable, so is yours. Minimize your wait time by arriving punctually, and by scheduling the first appointment at the beginning of your physician's day or the first appointment after lunch. If your doctor repeatedly keeps you waiting in the outer office, call in just before you leave your home or office to verify that he or she is running on schedule.

If you are trying to reach your doctor by phone, call the very first minute the office opens. In all likelihood, your physician will not be seeing a patient yet; he or she may be doing paper-work and preparing for patients who are scheduled to come in. If you don't get through, leave a message where you can be reached. Be sure to leave your home, office, and cell phone numbers, as doctors are rarely able to return calls immediately.

Here again, the more knowledgeable you are, the more effective your communications will be. Make certain that your physician has a complete treatment plan for you, not just a schedule of prescriptions. He or she also must be able to explain this plan to you. In the best of all worlds, you will want not only a treatment plan but to know what your physician's alternative plans are if one should become necessary. Prioritize and stream-line the process as much as you can.

The more time your doctor spends looking for information, the less time he or she will have for you. The more you help to organize your treatment, the easier it will be for your physician to keep things straight. Remember that keeping track of treatments is a challenge for your physician, just as it is for you. It has been estimated that paperwork adds at least thirty minutes to every hour of hands-on care provided for the average patient, and, in some settings, an hour to every hour of care.

GIVE TO YOUR HOSPITAL'S BLOOD BANK

Most blood banks are always running low because blood is such a precious substance and is always needed. Please try to give blood periodically, simply to help other people with medical problems. Specifically, however, you need to start giving blood the minute that the possibility of surgery is mentioned in your case. Blood donations from yourself and from your friends (even if they are not the same blood type) will assure that blood will be kept on reserve for you should surgery be necessary.

ALWAYS TRY TO CONSIDER YOUR DOCTOR'S SITUATION

In this and every other area, it is imperative that you try to understand your physician's position. This does not mean, however, that you should not be assertive in making your desires known and having your questions answered. Take notes; consider bringing a tape recorder on your visits. If possible, bring your designated health care advocate or a friend. There are many instances when the mere sight of a tape recorder or an advocate will inspire a physician to be in top form.

The physician who is strictly business oriented presents another kind of challenge. He or she wants you to be in and out of the office as soon as possible and may not be interested in your condition outside of the examination room. This is not Dr. Right. However, if you must deal with such physicians, challenge them on their own terms by coming prepared with your list of questions. Cut the small talk: bring your home situation into the conversation only if it affects your medical condition. Speak to them in plain, matter-of-fact ways and keep them on target. Approximately one-third of all the physicians in this country today speak English as their second language. If a communication problem exists—perhaps English is *your* second language, or you suffer from hearing loss—for whatever reason, if you cannot understand what a physician is telling you, make certain that a nurse or other medical professional is present who will explain carefully what the doctor has said so that you understand.

ALWAYS BE PROACTIVE

In all your dealings with physicians, take the proactive role. If problems arise, talk to the person with whom you have the problem to see if it can be resolved. If the problem cannot be resolved between the two of you, call your insurance company's member-services department and explain the problem. Log the time and date of the conversation and the name of the person with whom you spoke; keep a record of everything that is said.

However protracted your negotiations with your insurance company or physician may become, you can still appeal your case to your state insurance commissioner, to your local and state medical societies, and to the many advocacy groups whose purpose is to help in such circumstances. *Families USA*, listed in the resources section in the back of this book, provides a list of state agencies regulating health care.

SET UP COMPREHENSIVE HEALTH CARE FINANCIAL FILES

To better facilitate this process and to see you through the journey ahead, I strongly recommend that you set up a logical filing system for all bills, receipts, insurance forms, diagnosis sheets, lab results, and other medical paperwork. Throw nothing away. Document each visit to a physician, each communication with an insurance company representative, and all follow-up visits. Keep a separate log of all physicians, consultants, medical testing personnel, and laboratories that bill for services in your case. Make certain that you leave a long trail at each step along the way, and have ready access to it. This should not be just a paper trail, it should be an e-trail as well. Much information between doctors and insurers is now transmitted electronically. Ask your physician or specialist to copy you on correspondence—written or electronic—with your insurance carrier. If your physician believes in the diagnosis he or she has made, and the treatment prescribed, he or she ought to be willing to back it up in writing, explaining why the treatment is medically necessary. He or she should also be able to cite medical articles and references in support of that position—which you will also want to keep in your files.

AN IMPORTANT PIECE OF PAPERWORK

Among many useful pieces of paper you will need to have in your health care portfolio, perhaps the most important is the Very Necessary Medical Identification Card that you will find on page 249. This card will contain vital information for you in an emergency situation that can easily save you so much time and will correctly detail your current diagnosis, blood type, medicines you are taking, and notes on your known allergies. The card will also contain contact information for your doctor as well as insurance information, so that you do not have to carry as many papers when you go to medical appointments. This card can be a huge time-saver in both emergency and non-emergency situations. Please fill it out, laminate it, and keep it in your purse or wallet.

THE SOONER YOU CAN GET SUCH A SYSTEM in place, the easier it will be to appeal an insurance exclusion or get reimbursement for out-of-pocket expenses. In the rare event that you have grounds for filing a malpractice suit against your doctor, hospital, or both, you will have a much easier time substantiating your claims and position. At the very least it will be helpful in sorting out which bills you are responsible for paying and which belong to your insurance company. These same files will also be used to help you identify overcharges and other mistakes made in the billing process. They are more common than you might expect. A recent study found that up to 20 percent of hospital bills contain errors, most often in overcharges or charges for services never performed.

ADD A FILE OF QUESTIONS — AND ANSWERS

In addition to the files you will want to keep on all financial matters, medical personnel, and insurance claims will be files that list the many questions that you want answered. Depending on your condition and insurance coverage, you may choose to divide this file into categories, such as those questions you put to your insurance representative and those to your physicians and other health care providers. Foremost on this list will be the questions pertaining to your disease. You may wish to include answers given and the dates when those answers were provided.

NEVER STOP ASKING QUESTIONS

This section has given you some concept of how difficult and complicated the health care establishment can be. I hope that I have also provided you with sound advice about how to bring this monster under control. My advice is by no means comprehensive, and there are many other areas to consider, depending on your specific situation. Never stop asking questions and never fail to assert your rights if a financial situation seems problematic. Because whether you are very poor or very rich, it makes no difference in health care. If you continue to press your case, you can get the best health care available. Remember, you have only one life to live.

If you have health problems in addition to chronic illness or disease—problems such as smoking or substance abuse—you will want to ask whether your insurance plan offers smoking cessation, weight loss, or other benefits targeted to your needs. (Requests for medical help with your addictions can be a double-edged sword, however. If you admit to having these addictions, there is a good chance that the cost of your health insurance will be increased. Also, if you have a drug or alcohol addiction and are not covered by a company health policy, it is very costly, if not impossible, to obtain medical coverage until you can prove that you have been sober for seven to ten years.) If you want to seek out alternative medical treatment, you need to ask whether your plan will pay for it, and which specific treatments and kinds of doctors are covered. A high percentage of PPOs and HMOs cover chiropractic visits; considerably fewer cover acupuncture and homeopathy.

The support staff in your physician's office should be able to assist you in understanding what your policy provides and what it doesn't. If you are receiving service in a hospital, you can consult their patient advocate. All hospitals have them. Another good way to familiarize yourself with your policy is to request the help of the one of many organizations that have been established for this very purpose. These are the same groups that you will wish to consult in the event of problems stemming from insurance coverage, debt management, and other crises arising from medical care. The Patient Advocate Foundation, a nonprofit group created to help in such events, can be found on the Internet or contacted using a toll-free number. This information, as well as other helpful contacts, can be found in the resources section at the back of this book.

Step Nine Summary

1. Knowledge is power. Study and understand your insurance coverage, whether it is from an HMO, a PPO, a POS, or Medicare or Medicaid.
2. Become familiar with the peculiar language of the medical world. Doctors will use a lot of Latin phrases and other professionals will use acronyms, code numbers, and phrases that you need to know.
3. Set up a meeting with your doctor's billing administrator to discuss the best ways to coordinate and streamline insurance reimbursements and payments to labs, hospitals, other specialists—and, of course, to your doctor. Discuss how the medical coding system works in your doctor's office.
4. Make an appointment to meet the hospital administrator in the hospital where your doctor and specialists practice. You will want to make a friend for the future and to learn as much as you can about the complicated problems of hospital billing.
5. As you meet with your doctor over the course of treatment, make him or her a partner in both your healing and your health care finances. Working with the billing administrator, your doctor can create a win-win situation for you and for himself or herself while taming the monster.
6. Set up a separate and comprehensive filing system for your medical records and bills. Make detailed notes of every conversation, both in person and on the telephone. A thorough paper trail will serve you well in taming the monster.
7. Establish a monthly meeting with your accountant or financial adviser to review the status of all expenditures

related to your health care and recovery. Educating yourself means everything, and you need to have updated information about where your money is going.

8. Even after you feel you have good working relationships, excellent accounting systems, and reliable people to keep you updated on your finances, never relax your guard. Continue to ask questions. Make a separate file or journal for your questions—and the answers you are given.

STEP TEN

Give Back

THIS FINAL STEP in your journey to better health is especially meaningful because you will have come full circle to help others. Even more remarkable, you will discover that your efforts for others will be a restorative part of your own cure. I cannot explain why it works this way, but it has for me and many others. You will never experience any greater sense of euphoria than you will when you know that you have positively affected someone's life. All you need to do is stand up and be counted.

In this step, I will share my experiences in forming my Center Without Walls foundation and creating a successful fund-raising vehicle to support it, the RACE to Erase MS. I recognize that not everyone can or wants to do a grand-scale gala, but whatever love or talent you have, I hope that elements of my experience will be useful to you in giving back in many different ways. I will tell you about the amazing efforts of other people who have created foundations or fund-raising events of their own to combat many different diseases. At the heart of this step is the spirit of volunteerism, and I will explore some of the many ways anyone can volunteer at various levels. Finally, I want to tell you about how much my life has changed for the better after working through these steps—and assure you that yours will, too.

In your hands you hold the power to promote your recovery, share dietary and health tips, test the limits of standard medical treatments, explore alternative health therapies, and, by example, encourage others who have chronic illness or disease to do the same. I joined the legion of people who have gone a step further. This is the tenth step that I urge you to take. After getting over the initial shock of my diagnosis and seeing how it affected my body, I set out to find a cure for MS. I knew in my heart that I could not live with so little hope; I also knew that there were millions suffering the same frustrations I was.

I was truly lucky and also keenly aware that this was not the case for everyone. This is why I feel compelled to fight for others as well as myself. I knew then that there was a better answer than the prognosis I was offered. I felt I had no choice but to find a way to be healthy and live a normal life, because I was a young mother of three and could not bear the thought of my precious boys suffering and living their lives without a mother to be strong for them, to teach them, to be an active part of their lives. I could not stand for anybody to feel sorry for me, especially my children, whom I was fortunate to give life to. The thought of them having to grow up and push me around in a wheelchair was my motivation for truly fighting a fight and garnering a strength I'd never known I possessed.

The death-sentence diagnosis became a blessing in disguise, because it challenged me to become a much more evolved person, to test myself in ways I'd never dreamed possible, and to take charge of my life in ways I had never been able to previously. It gave me a career, one I never took courses for in college. As I developed a plan for myself, I realized that I had found a larger purpose to my life—to help others affected by any potentially devastating disease. There is truly no greater high or sense of satisfaction you can have than realizing that you have positively affected someone's life.

HELPING OTHERS IS A FINAL STEP IN RECOVERY

Similar to the twelve-step programs that have been useful for problems ranging from alcoholism to overeating, this final step in your progression to health is to share your experience with others and truly reach out to help those afflicted with your disease. Whether you have fully recovered or are still on the road to recovery, you have valuable insight to offer others who are just experiencing their initial shock. Much of this chapter is based on my experience of devoting a large part of my life to establishing a research foundation to fight multiple sclerosis and to raising money to support that fight. I can tell you from personal knowledge that giving back is not only rewarding, it is part of the cure—and a key to sustaining better health.

I feel as though I have taken on this disease in every way I know how, and now I am helping others to fight it, too. Together, we all are going to win. I am confident.

The Center Without Walls and the RACE to Erase MS were created out of a genuine desire to help others and to find a cure for MS. However, this process of giving back has transformed me. I am stronger, smarter, and healthier because of sharing. There is certainly no logical or scientific explanation for why this works for me and for millions of others, but it does.

CHALLENGE THE SYSTEM
TO FIND OPTIONS

In the years since I was diagnosed, I have challenged the system—especially doctors and others who presented multiple sclerosis as the end of my life—to find viable options for people with MS. The Center Without Walls is a unique national collaboration of the nation's top seven MS doctors, linking data, research, and results from the most prestigious medical centers: Harvard; the University of Southern California; the University of California, San Francisco; The Cleveland Clinic; Yale; Johns Hopkins; and the Oregon Health & Science University.

When I first envisioned this group of doctors working together in The Center Without Walls (CWOW), I was met with comments such as "You're out of your mind!" and "You don't know what you're talking about!" and "This can't be done!" I asked why and was always given the empty, pointless answer—that it wasn't traditional. My answer, of course, was that their traditions for the past fifty years had produced no known cure, no therapies, and no information to help people with multiple sclerosis. It was time to throw all traditions out the door.

Also what I found on my journey to locate the best doctors and researchers in the MS field was that they were all working on very important research studies and each thought that he or she was the only one doing that incredible study. When I would go to other doctors at other highly reputed medical centers, they were doing what appeared to be almost the identical study, but no one was communicating. That was when a light went on in my head and I realized what I had to do. Now, amazingly, doctors from seven medical centers around the country teleconference once a month and meet face-to-face four times a year with an energy and spirit that comes from the best and the brightest MS medical researchers in the world co-operating, communicating, and working together—not competing.

Together, they are working seven times faster to find a cure for MS. I truly honor this remarkable team of seven brilliant doctors for taking down the traditional barriers that exist in research and coming together to work as a team to truly fight MS. By reporting the negative research as well as the positive, other doctors creating new studies are armed with so much information about whether a drug dose is too high or too low or has some terrible side effect. It is imperative for doctors to communicate. It makes common sense if we ever hope to find cures for the horrendous diseases that plague us and the people we love.

I am especially proud of my work for CWOW. We have fundamentally changed the way MS research is conducted in the United States. CWOW has also helped to give direction to grassroots efforts that are taking place nationwide as like-minded teams of physicians, specialists, and researchers come together to share their expertise and insights.

Of course, medical research is expensive. I knew that I could not fund it alone, but I also knew that I had the skills to create a fund-raising event that could. In 1993, I conceived what has become the annual RACE to Erase MS, a celebrity ski event on the very slopes where my ski accident triggered the events that changed my life. It is now an annual event in Los Angeles that always has a special fashion show and musical theme.

I direct this event with my great friend and partner Tommy Hilfiger. Over its twelve-year history, friends, athletes, celebrities, and corporate sponsors have pitched in to raise more than $25 million. When we do an event, we are able to have almost every single cost underwritten by amazing and generous friends—including the event location, the flowers, the liquor, the invitations, the journal books, and even the "goody bags."

Ninety to ninety-five percent of the money raised (many charity events put in barely 25 percent of what they make, because
of extremely high expenses) goes directly to support the
groundbreaking MS research of The Center Without Walls.

The very first year of my event, I was lucky enough to meet
Tommy Hilfiger. He was the most fun and innovative man who
had a sister also suffering from MS. As his success grew, his gen-
erosity grew and he helped underwrite parts of the event and
even got VH1 to be our partner and air it for three years. Every
year, we sit down to create a new musical theme for our event.
Tommy is so creative and truly enjoys the process of giving
birth year after year to a completely different idea. He carries
the theme through and designs the most breathtaking invitations, produces the most energetic and stylish celebrity fashion
show, helps with giving us goody bags filled to the brim with
fabulous items, and always makes a generous donation on top of
that.

We always need to fly in entertainers and doctors from all
over the country, which can be very costly. For the last ten
years, American Airlines has been so generous to underwrite
this huge cost and also gives us another ten trips for all over the
world to our auction, which nets a lot more money for us.

Our entertainers always donate their time and talent, which
is a key part of our event. Over the years, we have been lucky to
have such stellar entertainers as Natalie Cole, Earth, Wind and
Fire, Don Henley, Stevie Nicks, No Doubt, Kate Bush, Stevie
Wonder, Kenny G, Donna Summer, the Goo-Goo Dolls, Cyndi
Lauper, and Michael Bolton. My dear friends Suzanne de Passe
and David Foster, true legends in the music business, have donated their time and talent to produce this event.

The most sought-after florist in Los Angeles, Mark's Garden, always creates the most breathtaking flower arrangements
to match the themes of our events each year.

Many of the drug companies that make MS drugs support us very generously. In 2004, Serono, Inc. helped us to publish a comprehensive booklet on MS that was sent to every doctor in the United States to educate them about every aspect of MS.

MAKE SURE YOU KNOW EXACTLY WHERE YOUR MONEY GOES

Starting your own group or joining another may not be the way you want to give of your resources. Dollars and cents may be the way you wish to contribute. Millions of Americans give generously every year. In fact, the $248.5 billion given to the top 400 charities in 2004 was an 11.6 percent increase over 2003. Do your homework. Go beyond the glossy charity brochure and make sure that the dollars you give are targeted for your intended goal. Look for the line item costs. Make it a rule to find out what percentage of dollars donated to a particular cause actually goes into research, and how much goes to overhead, administration, and fund-raising. It's easy to feel good about giving, but it's even better to know that your giving will actually reach the people for whom it was intended.

As ridiculous as this may sound, most of the money you raise for charity will not go where you think it is going. Most of the time, about 90 percent of the money won't go where you think it is going unless you really go the extra mile. People work so hard and put in so many hours to create the perfect event and afterward you always see these gigantic-check-signing ceremonies. But that is just when the hard work begins. The truth is that it is just as hard to spend the money correctly as it is to raise it. It is critical that you meet with the doctors or hospitals who are the recipients of your fund-raisers and ask them where they are most in need of your donation—where it will make the biggest difference. After you mutually decide on this you must request the doctors to make a budget for the project for one year or—ideally—fill out an NIH grant form. At least, you must ask them to provide a detailed letter that breaks down how much goes to each item, including the doctors' and other researchers' time, lab work, and other data.

If you simply give unrestricted money, you can be sure that your donated dollars will not go where you think they should. Doctors and hospitals have so many people they treat who are not paying for their blood work or X-rays or appointments. There is a large chance that your money will fill in these blanks for them and not affect positive change in the area you most care about. Early on, when deciding where this hard-earned money should go, I learned about a very common practice in university-associated hospitals called a "chancellor's fee." This means that whatever you donated to the hospital, 10 percent automatically came off the top, which most people were never made aware of. What exactly is a chancellor's fee? This money goes to fund the college chancellor's home, travel, and entertainment budget. You may be paying for caviar and champagne parties, instead of affecting change in diseases such as cancer, AIDS, and heart disease. I was told with the universities to which we were donating, there was simply nothing I could do about that. It was, again, a "tradition." I then refused to give money to anyone who would take even a dime for a chancellor's fee. Funny enough, we were soon able to give money entirely to the cause and not support the chancellor's activities.

Every year, the doctors at all seven members of The Center Without Walls submit an NIH grant form. This is a very lengthy and difficult task, but it shows you the importance and goal of the work and details exactly what it will cost for a year, between lab supplies, MRIs, and doctors' salaries. The form requires doctors to provide a breakdown of the percentage of their time that they will commit to the project. After we receive all these proposals, they are reviewed and graded by our scientific advisory board, a group of very bright and talented doctors who are not associated with the hospitals or medical centers we fund directly. Their judgments are completely fair and unbiased. We have had to reject proposals and drop those applicants who did not rate a 1 or a 2 on an NIH Grant Scale of 1 to 5. I would never work this hard raising money only to have it go to mediocre research.

THE ROOTS OF MY FUND-RAISING EXPERIENCE

I was first presented with the importance of creating charity events when my sister, at age seven, was diagnosed with juvenile diabetes. I was away for my freshman year of college and had just come home for Thanksgiving vacation. I was so excited to return for the first time. When I sat down at the dinner table expecting everybody to be happy to see me, there was an eerie silence and everyone looked very downcast. When I asked what was wrong, nobody would talk. A sea of tears began to roll down the faces of my mother, father, and younger brother. My seven-year-old sister bravely offered that she had "diadeedes." That, of course, was followed by the most intense and sorrowful explanation of my sister's disease.

Childhood diabetes is incurable and she would have to live with it for the rest of her life. In the next few days, I also learned of the devastating side effects, such as blindness and loss of limbs. I sat with my sister as she had blood tests and shots that would terrify any child, but especially one who had to have at least three a day just to keep alive. I looked at my little sister as the most beautiful and perfect princess and I could not bear for her to suffer.

My mother, Barbara Davis, was devastated and was never

one to take "no" for an answer, especially when it came to her family. She knew that she was enormously lucky to have the resources to take Dana to the best diabetes doctors our country had to offer, which at the time was at the Joslin Clinic in Boston. Where we lived, in Colorado, and within a five-state region, there was no hospital or comprehensive center to treat children with diabetes and their whole families. Soon, my mother created an event to build what is now called the Barbara Davis Center for Childhood Diabetes, in Denver.

She called her fund-raising event the Carousel Ball, and that was where I learned how to organize a charity event. I was in charge of the silent auction. We used to have meetings in my living room asking all of our friends and volunteers to come up with unique auction ideas and help us secure them. At this time, nobody was doing silent auctions. As the chair, I felt so excited at how easy it was to get an amazing array of auction items, and the amount we made was earth-shattering, while having little or no expenses. It gave me such a great feeling inside, seeing how getting great auction items could translate into a potential cure for children's diabetes so that my little sister would not have to suffer.

Mom, of course, worked tirelessly and created one of the most successful fund-raisers that exists in our country to this day. Unfortunately, a cure for diabetes has still not been discovered, but so much was found to help everybody living with this devastating disease. They have a prolonged and better quality of life. Everything started at a very grass-roots level with friends all giving from their hearts, and the event has attracted the most respected doctors in our country. When I was diagnosed with MS, this training gave me the insight and discipline to know that I had an important mission to accomplish. In my heart, I had to start the RACE to Erase MS.

The focus of much of my work has been on foundation development and management, fund-raising and event planning, and on facilitating a greater understanding of how public health policy is shaped by government and the private sector. I want to fund many basic science projects in different areas of MS and be sure that the researchers are constantly communicating and never duplicating their efforts.

I am not alone. Hundreds, perhaps thousands of disease-awareness and fund-raising organizations have begun in much the same way as my own. In 1980, Nancy Brinker lost her sister, Susan Goodman Komen, to breast cancer. Nancy was then a thirty-six-year-old mother of two young children. As she watched her sister die, she wondered how this could happen in one of the most medically advanced countries in the world. Nancy promised Susan that she would dedicate the rest of her life to eradicating breast cancer as a life-threatening disease. Two years later, Nancy Brinker established the Susan G. Komen Breast Cancer Foundation with only a few hundred dollars of her own and a shoebox full of index cards.

This was before Nancy herself discovered that she had breast cancer. Today, her foundation is the largest private funder of breast cancer research in the nation. Under her leadership, the foundation has raised more than $27.5 million and has awarded more than two hundred research grants.

GIVING BACK COMES IN ALL SHAPES AND SIZES

Disease-awareness and fund-raising groups come in all shapes and varieties. One of the most remarkable examples of raising awareness that I know about is the movie *Lorenzo's Oil*, which was released in 1992, with Susan Sarandon, Nick Nolte, and Peter Ustinov. It was directed and cowritten (with Nick Enright) by George Miller, an M.D. This is a fictional story based on the real lives of Michaela and Augusto Odone, whose son, Lorenzo, was diagnosed with adrenoleukodystrophy (ALD) at age five. The Odones were told, as I was, that there was no cure, no hope. As I did, they ignored the negativity and began to educate themselves about ALD. Despite opposition from the medical establishment, they concluded that, similar to MS, ALD is caused by the deterioration of the myelin sheath that protects neurons in the human nervous system. This, in turn, causes eventual loss of sight, hearing, speech, ambulation—and eventual death.

The Odones found that the deterioration of the myelin was due to a buildup of saturated fatty acids that caused the sheath to dissolve. To counter the damage of saturated fatty acids, they developed a blend of unsaturated oils derived from plants that seems to block the myelin damage and to reduce ALD symptoms. Dubbed "Lorenzo's Oil," the substance is four parts oleic acid and one part erucic acid.

The film hit a nerve in me. I realized that no one else was going to rush to discover "Nancy's Oil"; that was going to be my job. Don't assume that things will just drop into your lap.

Although ALD patients typically die within a few years of diagnosis. Lorenzo is still alive at age twenty-seven in mid-2005. His father, Augusto, heads the Myelin Foundation in Washington, D.C., where research based on Lorenzo's Oil continues to show promise in both laboratory and clinical tests.

The Texas Neurofibromatosis Foundation was founded in 1980 by an Austin woman whose son had NF, a genetic disorder that causes disfiguring tumors. Most people back then did not know of the disease, partially because people who have it tend to shield themselves to avoid public ridicule. During the ten years after it was founded, the families involved with the foundation led a grass-roots campaign to raise money from walkathons, skateathons, garage sales, and a crawfish festival. An annual golf tournament was established to support a small office in Austin, Texas, which raised funds to support budding research projects.

The Neurofibromatosis Foundation has been a group of highly motivated and energetic volunteers eager to share their time and resources. Often the beginnings of such groups are modest. Some groups are formed by celebrities after they or someone they love has been diagnosed with an "incurable" disease. Richard Richards was a promising young baseball player when he lost his arm to neurosarcoma. Today he runs *The Men's Forum*, a television interview program that explores men's health produced at Rogue Valley Community Television in Ashland, Oregon. Television personality Leeza Gibbons started her own foundation after her mother was diagnosed with Alzheimer's. Leeza's Place today consists of a network of drop-in centers that offer safe haven for those with any type of memory disorder, where caregivers and loved ones get education as they adjust to their new reality.

HEAL YOURSELF AND HEAL OTHERS, TOO

Carol Eustice was a nineteen-year-old college student when she was diagnosed with rheumatoid arthritis. Today she uses her thirty years of personal experience with a variety of treatments, medications, and joint surgeries to counsel and moderate the weekly "Rheumatoid Arthritis Chat Group" on AOL. Marion Woodman was diagnosed with cancer and was told that she had two months to live. She and her husband went out to a graveyard to choose a plot, but today she heads an educational foundation dedicated to teaching techniques for uniting the mind, body, and spirit into a healing force. In healing themselves, these people have helped to heal many others.

The recipe for these individual successes rests in the spirit of leadership. They have exemplified that key element in the recovery process: gratitude for being given an opportunity to heal themselves. They have a passion for appreciating a life that could so easily have been ruled out. They look past obstacles and view things as possible. They have found ways to break through the barrier of naysayers and pessimists. They see themselves and the world around them in a positive light. Their leadership serves as examples for all of us.

THE HEALING POWER OF GIVING

After my event every year, feeling totally spent and exhausted, not seeing how I could possibly do an event the next year, I always receive the most amazing letters and phone calls from those who suffer from multiple sclerosis, telling me what a big difference I have made in their lives. There is no greater high or sense of euphoria than truly believing that you have the power to affect positively someone's health and entire life. It always encourages me to start planning my next event immediately, and to fight even harder. I truly feel that by working so hard to cure MS, my health is ten times better than it would be. Although it makes no sense, I feel that all those endless hours of work on all things MS gives me a pass for good health.

Much has been said about the positive ripple effect that such good work has brought into the world. There is one aspect, however, that generally goes unmentioned: the healing power of living a life dedicated to raising the consciousness of others. The encouragement these people provide to others with illnesses cannot be measured in traditional terms. It is not only psychological, it is physiological. As modern science now knows, the positive reinforcement that comes from receiving encouragement actually stimulates neurotransmitters in the brain. This enhances energy levels, powers of creativity, and endurance. It is something that professional sports coaches have known for years. Inspirational leaders bring out the best in us.

From the very first event I held in Aspen, I learned how amazing it was to touch the lives of others. I lacked confidence doing my first event. I went on a radio talk show in Aspen to tell my personal story with MS. I did not realize how telling my story, as embarrassing as that sometimes is, has far-reaching effects.

The next day I had a volunteer meeting and quickly noticed a young woman in a wheelchair being wheeled in by her mother. After this meeting was over, they came up to me with big tears in their eyes and simply said thank you. I said, "Thank you for what?" The mother said, "My daughter heard you on the radio last night. She is your same age, was diagnosed when you were, has children the same age as your children, and was told what you were told: to go home and go to bed. She listened to the doctors and you didn't. You really hit a nerve with her. She hasn't gotten dressed or left her home in two years. She is sad, depressed, and hasn't really taken care of her kids or really participated in her marriage in that time. When she heard you, she could really relate. She got dressed in clothing today for the first time, and look at her ears: she is wearing earrings!"

I got very choked up, and at that moment I understood that what I had to say and do for MS really did matter and was far-reaching. Anybody can do this and realize how powerful anything they do to help a cause really is. We immediately helped her to see the right doctors and her health was finally going in a positive direction with hope—hope that she had finally found.

The experience of dealing with chronic illness and disease has given all of us a rare opportunity to serve others by giving them our best, by setting an example, and by going the extra distance necessary to make a difference in our world. There are many small and large ways we can serve one another. Any contribution you can make in any way, shape, or form is more valuable than anything you can do.

THE SPIRIT OF VOLUNTEERISM

I advocate volunteerism, which was the way I was raised. Today, our nation is the world leader in volunteerism. Last year, 28 percent of Americans—more than 64 million people—worked without pay for causes ranging from legal aid to flood relief to physical therapy. No matter what your age or condition, I urge you to join their ranks. Your insights, skills, and depth of character that have led you on the journey to recovery will be a symbol of hope for those who will follow.

The easiest way to get started is to recognize the opportunities in the many outreach programs, volunteer service organizations, and charities that exist in areas of interest to you. Not everyone needs to start a charity or research center. Just being involved with like-minded people with shared goals will have the benefit of keeping you from becoming isolated. I urge you, however, to go the extra distance and make your mission larger than just yourself. Never feel intimidated that you do not have enough pull, creativity, time, or money. Whatever you can do is truly meaningful.

To prepare for volunteer work, first you must make a self-assessment. In addition to giving back, ask yourself what your real motivations are for volunteering.

FINDING A GOOD FIT

If you have asked yourself a few honest questions about what you want as a volunteer, you now need to look at what you have to offer and how that may fit with what different organizations need:

- At the very least, you have experience as a person who is fighting or has a loved one fighting a life-altering disease. That experience will give you insights and empathies to share with others that may be unique. It will also give you the raw emotional energy you need to conquer that disease.
- If you enjoy meeting others, you may wish to volunteer as a door-to-door fund-raiser or as a support-group organizer.
- If communications is your skill, you can help with newsletters, letter writing, or media campaigns.
- People with computer skills are particularly in demand. There are a wide variety of ways you can contribute by researching so many important factors and putting them together.
- Assess your time. Decide if you can offer an organization particular times on weekends or regular spots on weekdays. Perhaps you would prefer to fill spots that would allow you to work at a telephone or a computer station at your own pace.
- Do not be afraid to shop around. Find an organization that is right for you and stands for what you stand for.
- Make sure the money you are helping to raise is truly being spent in its intended place. This is much harder to do than you might expect. Do your research and make sure every question you have is answered.
- You can also volunteer your time to work in a hospital or nursing home.

SURVEY THE GROUPS AND SERVICES IN YOUR COMMUNITY

Do your homework. Find out which groups already exist in your community that share your goals. The hospitals you've been to and the Internet sites you've visited are good places to start looking, as are community centers and health service newsletters. If you are considering starting your own group, look around first. Duplication of efforts hurts new and old organizations alike by competing for public attention and scarce financial resources—to the extent that both may fail. If you find one or more groups dealing with your issues already in place, talk with those who participate and try to find common ground. See what unique ideas or talent you can bring to the table.

When I was diagnosed with MS, I was approached by an MS organization that acted as though they had hit lotto. They wanted to romance me to be on their board in the hope that I would give generously, build a building or something truly out of my reach. I studied where they were putting their money and was very unsatisfied. I knew in my heart that with their antiquated approach, they would never find a cure for MS. During their many years in existence they had raised hundreds of millions of dollars for research, with the result at that point of no known cause, no known cure, no therapies for MS, and no foreseeable future.

I knew from my experience working on the Carousel Ball that a grass-roots effort with lots of volunteers, a great plan to educate the public, and the greatest doctors working as a team and not competing, but consistently communicating, we had a much better chance to find a cure. I was met with much resistance in the beginning, but now it is a successful working model.

No matter what your disease or passion, it is important to find your niche. Listen to your heart, no matter what anybody tells you, get organized the best you know how, using every resource possible, and go after it. Do not listen to the naysayers. Do what you know is right. Do it now. Don't wait until you feel better. It just might be the thing that makes you gain your health back.

Having clearly defined objectives is an important first step. You may wish to invite groups of friends and supporters out for coffee or into your home to get started. The more relaxed the setting and the more lively the discussion, the more fun and rewarding it will be. Large or small, the purpose is to build bridges. It may take one meeting or fifty, but everyone participating in your group eventually must be able to give a realistic account of what the objectives of the organization will be. If you cannot clearly identify those objectives, go back to the drawing board. Potential new members must understand exactly what you are working to achieve, and what they will be asked to do.

YOUR ORGANIZATION IS A LIVING ENTITY

The organization should be considered a living entity, and, like all living things, it will grow and evolve over time. Update your database regularly. People's lives change—they move, divorce, remarry. Even your most dedicated supporters may not remember to let you know when they have new information. When your mailings are returned or that phone number is no longer in service, work on getting an update.

There will be many opportunities for increasing membership. One-on-one meetings with people are always the best method to educate others and bring them into the group. Information can be distributed in newsletters. The Internet and e-mail are also great resources, which I will discuss in more detail later in the resources section.

You will want to notify your community, first of the existence of your group, then of its ongoing activities. Here as elsewhere, the key to success is organization. Get the word out by linking up with a group that has sponsored an event, or by sharing booth space at a county fair or health expo. Partner with other advocates and community leaders who have shared interests and have demonstrated a commitment to your issue or similar issues. Enlisting the support of well-respected community leaders, elected officials, and candidates for public office can add credibility and visibility, as can allies such as business and industry leaders. I have had a great deal of assistance from celebrities who are willing to use their high profiles for good purposes. Do your homework and try to find one or more actors, actresses, sports figures, politicians, and other "local celebrities" willing to support your cause. Whatever city you live in, there is always a celebrity, one whom people admire and look up to. Honor them, have them come to your events, put their names on your invitations. It always helps because that translates into earning more money.

COMMUNICATE WELL AND LOOK FOR THE POSITIVE

People get involved and stay involved in an organization because they feel they can make a positive difference. As an organization grows, so do its bureaucratic structures. Do all you can to keep such structures from interfering with the team spirit. To feel appreciated, one must be appreciated. Share the success as you share the responsibilities. Don't let bureaucracy interfere with your goals. Always thank anyone and everyone over and over for anything they do to help your charity. In the back of your mind, you should always remember that they are not getting paid and don't have to do anything, and you always want to leave the door open for the next event you might do.

MAKE YOUR PASSION CONTAGIOUS

Whenever you plan an event, you want it to be unique, fun, and memorable. There are ways to put on the most amazing events and get almost everything underwritten. But you should never spend so much on food, decor, and flowers that you net less than 60 percent of what you make at the very least. Our event is able to net at least 90 percent. The first thing you need to do is apply for a tax ID number, better known as a 5o1c3. This way your organization is set up so that donations can be deductible.

Plan your event and see what you can possibly get donated. Call on those you frequently give business to—you might be surprised by how generous they are. If somebody shares the particular disease you are fighting, they might also want to give their product to you or give at a discounted rate.

Not everybody doing a charity event needs to do their work on a grand scale. Any idea you have that raises any amount of money for charity is truly important. Choose something that is fun for you or that you are excited about, something you have a talent for. Sometimes just the unusual ideas that have little or no expense might warrant the greatest amounts of money. The Lance Armstrong Foundation for cancer research authorized Nike to create yellow rubber bracelets that have LIVESTRONG imprinted on the face. Originally sold at a dollar each, resale values have been rocketing up since the original 10 million sold out. Everyone can afford to make a donation of that size and feel good about the cause. They are also now a fashion statement and everybody is now mimicking this idea in a variety of colors for different causes. If you are a runner, organize a small run and get donors to sponsor you per mile. Every year these types of events really grow.

Never look down on your ideas. Follow your passion and

never be afraid to try something new to help raise money to fight the disease you want to erase.

STAND UP AND BE COUNTED

The "lucky" opportunity you have been given is a chance to expand your horizons and those of the people with whom you come into contact. Not everybody has the expertise, training, and resources to undertake a large enterprise geared to global reform. Even if you feel that you do not have a talent or are not connected, know that anything you can do to help a charity—no matter how small or how large it is—is truly important. Every single person with a generous and giving mind-set is truly a saint, and all the different parts add up to one very powerful sum.

Each of us can join with others to lift the consciousness of the world, one person at a time. And all of us can tailor the opportunities that we have to fit our unique differences and individual circumstances.

There are no rules. If you share my desire to give back in a larger way, you might consider starting your own charity organization. Figure out how you might best share your recovery expertise and talents to help others overcome their fears and bring empowerment and hope. I believe that each of us has a very personal and dynamic role to play in removing the word *incurable* from the public's perception of illness and disease. This is what I wish for every person—no matter what his or her diagnosis. Together we can do something about it, and along the way, we can influence our future, and that of our children. Each of us must take responsibility for whatever we can do, even if it is giving back one-on-one or friend-to-friend.

My final piece of advice is also my first: Stand up and be counted. Thinking and doing are two different things. It's the "getting started" that makes the important difference. Make that call to the friend you heard shares your disease. Sharing the details of your recovery may be the first step in building the bridge that will make what you have done the most meaningful—for you and for everyone.

Step Ten Summary

1. There is a wide range of ways for you to give back.
2. Giving back is a part of your recovery. By helping to heal others, you heal yourself.
3. Volunteering is the American way; it is part of the fabric of our country.
4. Assess your skills and time to determine a good fit with organizations that may need your help.
5. You may want to establish your own foundation or organization to fight a disease or to support people who are struggling.
6. Leadership and communication are vital to a successful organization.
7. If you make donations, be sure that the money you give is really reaching the intended recipients and not ending up in the hands of professional fund-raisers.
8. Connect with your passion about a cause and your feelings will be contagious.

ER BASICS

Dr. Joel Geiderman, co-chair of the Cedars-Sinai Medical Center Department of Emergency Medicine, notes that although his facility is well-equipped and well-staffed—with three doctors onsite every night—they are operating at or near capacity virtually every day. "Some days, we have to divert emergency patients to other hospitals because we are overwhelmed," explains Dr. Geiderman. In Los Angeles, where I live, so many ERs have closed due to insurance problems that the remaining good ones are completely overcrowded. Approximately half the patients at Cedars-Sinai hospital—a medical facility that I, my family, and friends have used frequently—come through the ER, even though only 30 percent of the people who come to the ER are admitted to the hospital.

Many people do not understand that if you dial 911 in an emergency situation, you will not be given any choice of hospital. You will be taken to the nearest available ER by public am-

artment paramedic

s not have adequate

articular illness, you

ulance and request-

ou. This requires ad-

spital where you can

have that ER tele-

e in your house. You

a private ambulance

at you need.

ncy room visit. Read

overage regarding ER

nder contract to your

ER will be designated

u would be taken to if

home or office. They

it is and how to get

the ER unit, shop for

s to ask:

duty at any one time,

established hospital

g each shift, and how

onably accomodate in

me?

cial certifications?

na team?

at are their specialties?

d to handle your exact

cy on handling emer-

The answers to these questions will enable you to better determine the potential effectiveness of an ER unit. If the ratio of doctors to patients is greater than one doctor for every ten patients, or one nurse for every five patients, it may mean that the ER is understaffed. If the kind of specialist you anticipate needing is not on the list of specialists on call, you will want to know how the ER will address your needs. If you have a brain hemorrhage, for example, and there are no brain surgeons on call, you may be moved to another hospital—but which one, and how long might it take to transfer you there? In the event that you think your ER unit is understaffed or doesn't have the specialists suited to handle your particular needs, express your concern to your primary physician and your insurance carrier as soon as possible so that other arrangements can be made.

KNOW YOUR HEALTH CARE INSURER'S REQUIREMENTS REGARDING THE ER

Once you have chosen an ER that best meets your needs, find out what your insurance carrier's protocols are regarding that unit and what documentation you will have to provide when you arrive. In some cases—absurd as it may sound—you may be required to contact your insurance agent in advance of any ER visits. You may also have to make a co-payment when you get there, so you will want to be prepared with cash or a credit card. Keep all important documents, along with your need-to-know phone numbers, in a readily accessible file that you can take to the ER with you.

It is possible in these circumstances that you may not be conscious or able to communicate necessary information. This is when your health care advocate has to be nearby and educated about your issues. He or she must be ready to speak for you when you are not able.

re advocate what you
'our advocate should
policy information,
tions you are taking,
bers. (The Very Nec-
filled out is included
medical information
ur wallet or purse.)
or the ER physicians
gistration process. De-
have made with your
or she may be able to
nd have the ER staff

u will also want to be
ed and when it is not.
isits that are not true
. An unnecessary trip
gerous to your health.
xposure to viruses and
nproper diagnosis and

re chaos is created and
-rays being misplaced
tory. At the very least,
ay result in a six-hour
unately, ERs are over-
ot have urgent medical
for colds and minor ill-
dical insurance or the
s backs up the wait for

DO NOT WAIT: CALL 911

In the event that you are alone and judge yourself to be in a critical condition, your best option for immediate service is to call 911, the nationwide telephone emergency number for paramedics. Provide the dispatcher with as much information as possible, including your location, the type of emergency you have, and details of your condition. Stay on the line until the dispatcher tells you to hang up. Even if your condition turns out to be less urgent than you initially thought, in matters of life and death it is better to err on the side of caution.

There are several general rules that you will want to consider when calling 911 or a private ambulance service:

- You need or want medically trained personnel because of a possible back or neck injury.
- You need CPR (cardiopulmonary resuscitation) or oxygen.
- You are having convulsions or a seizure.
- You need help to stop the bleeding.

In the event that you decide your condition does not warrant calling 911, you can call for a private ambulance, have a friend drive you to the ER, go there by taxi, or accept a ride from someone on the spot. Know that if you come in an ambulance, you will be seen by a doctor much faster than if you come in on your own.

Paramedics may not be necessary:

- If you are in pain but are clearheaded.
- If the pain comes and goes.
- If you have experienced similar symptoms before and

know what treatment you need and know how soon you need it.

- If you have spoken to your doctor and he or she has told you that you do not need to call for an ambulance.

Never drive yourself to the ER if there is any danger of losing consciousness, if you are bleeding profusely, or if you are in severe pain. If you think you can drive yourself, it probably means that your condition is not sufficiently critical to warrant going to the ER. Call a taxi only as a last resort. There is no guarantee that a cab will arrive in a timely way or come at all.

Do not drink or eat while waiting, because this may interfere with treatment you may receive at the ER. Make certain that you have your medical records, insurance card, and other papers. Do not bring any valuables, pajamas, toiletries, extra clothes, or personal items. If all goes well, you may be home in a few hours. If you have to stay in the hospital, your health care advocate or someone from your support group can retrieve what you need.

Generally Accepted Reasons to Go to the ER:

- You have difficulty breathing or severe shortness of breath.
- Signs of a potential stroke.
- You lose consciousness or have been knocked out by a blow to the head.
- You have signs of a heart attack. Symptoms may include pain across the chest or under the breastbone, pain radiating outward or up from the chest, a sensation of squeezing or pressure in the chest.
- You suspect that you have had food poisoning.
- You are having a severe or worsening allergic reaction.

- You have suffered any major injury, especially one to the head or neck, or one that leaves you with blurry or double vision.
- Unexplained stupor, drowsiness, or disorientation.
- You have a broken bone or suspect you have a broken bone and your physician cannot see you the same day.
- You are experiencing severe abdominal pain.
- You are coughing up or vomiting blood.
- You are bleeding from a cut or wound that does not stop after ten minutes of direct pressure.
- You have received a wound that warrants receiving stitches.
- You have an unusually prolonged high fever.
- You have a possible drug overdose.
- You are in active labor.

In all of the above critical situations, use your best judgment and trust your instincts. If time permits, call your primary care physician and describe your symptoms. He or she may determine that urgent care is not necessary and may be willing to rearrange his or her schedule to see you in the office that same day. If ever possible during doctors' hours, it will normally be faster to go to your doctor's office, unless you are experiencing a critical emergency. Contacting your physician is a good idea in any event, because he or she may be willing to meet you at the ER, or at least call the ER in advance of your visit to inform them of your medical history. Your PCP may also indicate any special treatments or procedures you are receiving and any drug reactions you have had. Be sure that your physician or whoever answers the phone understands that your condition is critical. Make certain that you or whoever makes the call uses the word "emergency." If your doctor is unavailable, ask for an immediate callback, but don't put off going to the ER. If you have not heard

ve someone call your
office know that you
getting there.

EVALUATE
ON

iewed and examined
dge the seriousness of
Don't be disappointed
seen it on television
a single episode of ER
. Your vital signs will
, blood pressure, and

ke a proper diagnosis,

lem or condition first.
ou are, the more diffi-
ition.
ng you have had them,
d your visit.
or foods to which you

ant. Do not hold back
er how personal.
n your medical records,
taking, and especially
ification Card.

- If your health care advocate is present, allow him or her to take charge of providing the ER staff with the necessary information.
- Make certain that the ER staff calls your primary care physician. If you are being treated by specialists, they should be notified, too.
- Do not be afraid to ask questions. You or your health care provider must fully understand what is being said to you.

Registration usually takes place after the attending physician or nurse has examined you. This will not delay your treatment. In addition to filling out the paperwork regarding your insurance, you or your health care advocate will be presented with waivers that permit the ER staff to make emergency decisions and order X-rays and other diagnostic tests. This is standard procedure. If you and your advocate have done your homework, there should be no surprises or unexpected documents to sign.

The waiting period for ER treatment can be several minutes or an average of six hours, depending on the number of patients who have come in before you and the urgency of your need for medical intervention. If your vital signs are within normal limits and there is no sign of internal or external bleeding, you will most likely be assigned a lower priority level than patients whose injuries and illness are time-sensitive. Unfortunately, emergency rooms are crowded with adults and children who have no health insurance and no regular medical care. By federal law, emergency rooms are required to treat anyone who comes through their doors, regardless of their ability to pay. Thus emergency room waiting areas are busy all hours of the night and day and long waits are usual.

Triage Priority Levels
(from most critical to least critical):

- **Code:** This refers to someone who has suffered cardiac arrest outside of the hospital, or to someone whose vital signs crash within the emergency department. Most often, resuscitation efforts are already in progress before the patient has reached the hospital. The patient goes straight into the trauma room where an emergency team is standing by. In the event of a stroke, there are now anticlotting drugs, such as tPA (tissue plasminogen activator) that can be used to save brain tissue up to three hours after the first signs of a stroke. However, these drugs can cause abnormal bleeding and are considered dangerous if used after that short three-hour window.

- **Critical:** This designation denotes a person with stable vital signs who is exhibiting symptoms or has a history that clearly delineates a life-threatening condition. This might be a patient with chest pain, shortness of breath, and profuse sweating. In some cases, the nurse will administer initial treatment.

- **Urgent:** This designation describes patients with serious conditions that require medical intervention within two hours. These are people with abdominal pain, high fever, or other critical symptoms. They may have lacerations from a wound, but the bleeding is under control.

- **Nonurgent disabled:** These individuals are unable to walk or remain upright in a chair or whose condition has been determined that up to a four-hour wait is clinically acceptable.

- **Ambulatory:** This is a designation in which the nurse has determined that emergency care is not necessary. It describes people who have come in with colds, toothaches, headaches, bumps, bruises, abrasions, small lacerations, and skin rashes. They are usually the patients who wait the longest for care.

You or your health care advocate should ask what designation you have been given—this is especially important if you have been given a low priority. Ask the triage nurse why you have been given it. If you believe the designation is not correct, call the nursing supervisor. If you feel your symptoms have gotten worse, report it immediately and tell the supervising nurse that you feel your condition is deteriorating. Here, as elsewhere, you must be truthful. Don't exaggerate. Pretending you have passed out will not fool nurses and doctors, and if it does, you may receive the wrong treatment. As anxious as you might be from the long wait, do not berate the people checking you in. They are just doing their jobs and the kinder you are to them, the kinder they will be to you. Be persistent, but do not be rude.

GET THE EMERGENCY ATTENTION YOU REQUIRE

Once inside the ER treatment unit, you will likely be given blood and urine tests and hooked up to an IV. There may also be X-rays and MRIs. Such tests normally take only a brief time. X-rays, for example, can be shot and developed in ninety seconds; if there are delays, as there often are, you or your health care advocate should be told why. Do not allow your physicians or nurses to ignore your needs. If your symptoms have changed since your arrival at the ER, make certain that you report how severe they were at their worst. If you are feeling dizzy or are having vision problems, let them know. Remember: you didn't come to the ER to wait. It is an emergency.

In the event that you are not receiving the timely treatment you believe is required, there are several options available to you. You can sit and wait patiently, trusting the ER staff to address your condition after the more urgent cases have been attended to. Your health care advocate can go back to the triage nurse and be more forceful about your need for treatment. Use terms, if true, that you know will get a response: "I'm having trouble breathing," "the pain is intense," "I'm losing consciousness," and "I can no longer move my head or neck fully."

Although your ER has a responsibility to treat you in a timely way, you too have obligations. The ER staff's effectiveness depends on your cooperation. Follow the instructions you are given. Do not complain or resist if your clothes are removed or cut away. If your nurse or physician wants you to wear a neck brace, let them put it on and don't remove it unless you are directed to do so. If you are asked to undress and put on a hospital gown—the kind that ties in the back—do as you are told. This will make your physicians' work much easier. They are highly skilled professionals. Let them do their jobs.

Once the results from your tests are received, the doctor will explain them to you. More testing may be necessary. The treatment you receive may be simple or complex. It may take minutes or hours. It will be up to the supervising physician to recommend whether you can be discharged from ER or whether you need to be admitted to the hospital. Each hospital will have its own policy regarding your discharge. Regardless of what they say, however, the ultimate decision about whether you are ready to leave rests with you. Do not permit yourself to be released unless you are confident that the emergency is over.

If a life-threatening situation presents itself and you are unable to speak for yourself or have someone speak on your behalf, it is necessary to have a Very Necessary Medical ID Card in your wallet or on your person. The vital information about your current medical condition, doctors treating you, any drug or food allergies, and more about your personal medical history that is printed on this card just might save your life.

VERY NECESSARY
MEDICAL IDENTIFICATION CARD™

Name _____

Address _____

Telephone Numbers _____

Name and Telephone Number of Friend or Relative for Emergencies

_____

Date of Birth _____

Allergies _____

Blood Type _____

Current Illness _____

Past Illnesses _____

Name and Telephone Numbers of Your Primary Care Physician and Specialist_____

Name, Telephone Number, and ID Number of Health Care Insurer

_____

Do You Wish to Be an Organ Donor? _____

Please go to www.vnmedical-idcard.com to get information on how to order your Very Necessary Medical ID Card.

_____

_____

ELECTRONIC
HEALTH RESOURCES

The leading health care consumer site on the Internet is www.WebMD.com with 20 million visitors every month. This site offers carefully documented information and advice about all medical issues. In addition to excellent chat rooms for affinity groups and medical news, this service also features Medscape, which offers advanced information for doctors and other health care professionals with up-to-date news bulletins on medical research, as well as access to one hundred medical journals.

A helpful Internet site for information and resources for people with chronic illness or disease is www.healingwell.com. This site also provides access to chat rooms and discussion groups targeted specifically to particular illnesses and conditions. There are over fifteen hundred resources indexed here.

A good Web site that contains many interesting articles and resources for the chronically ill is run by the National Chronic

Care Consortium. They can be found on the Internet at
www.nccconline.org.

Another good all-around Web site is the Patients Guide to
Healthcare Information on the Internet, which can be found at
www.pslgroup.com/dg/c883a.htm.

Two physician-run Web sites containing much useful infor-
mation and important links to other sites are former Surgeon
General Dr. Koop's site at www.drkoop.com and Dr. Dean
Edell's site at www.healthcentral.com.

Much new research on medical breakthroughs can be found
through Medscape (a division of WebMD), which can be found
at www.medscape.com.

One of the best hospital Web sites is that of the Mayo
Clinic, which can be found at www.mayoclinic.com.

Information on specific diseases, treatments, health related
organizations, and health topics can be found at www.health
finder.gov.

Another good Web site for information on specific diseases
is Ask Noah, operated by New York Online Access to Health,
found at www.noah-health.org.

PubMed, a service of the National Library of Medicine, is a
good source for up-to-date biomedical information and has
links to many sites providing full text articles and other related
resources. They can be found at www.ncbi.nlm.nih.gov/
entrez/query.fcgi.

The National Guideline Clearinghouse, at www.guideline
.gov, is a great source for obtaining objective, detailed information on clinical practice guidelines.

A helpful Internet site for techniques for coping with
chronic illness and diseases is www.eldercareadvocates.com/
pages/art22.htm.

The *American Medical Association Directory of Physicians in
the U.S.* is a good multivolume set published by the AMA,

which lists names and credentials of every physician in the United States. This information is best accessed on the Internet at www.ama-assn.org.

The American Board of Medical Specialists directory of board-certified medical specialists has another multivolume set of books that lists board-certified U.S. and Canadian physicians and includes information on specialty, when certified, medical school and year of degree, place and dates of internship, and other information. They can be found at www .abms.org or by calling toll-free 866-275-ABMS.

The Public Citizen Health Research Group, founded by Ralph Nader in 1971, publishes a three-volume set of books that lists doctors who have been disciplined by state or federal agencies for incompetence, negligence, substance abuse, patient abuses, or the inappropriate distribution of prescription drugs. Check the reference section of your library, call 202-588-1000, or find them on the Internet at www .citizen.org.

The best database for information on physicians who have been involved in medical malpractice cases is the National Practitioner Data Bank (NPDB). This is currently closed to the lay public, but your attorney or health practitioner may be able to gain access to it. This database keeps a record of physicians who have been disciplined by medical boards or professional societies, paid on malpractice suits, and/or had hospital privileges suspended for more than thirty days. In some cases this same information can be obtained through the Public Citizen Health Research Group, a nonprofit organization that publishes a multivolume directory of doctors who have been disciplined. The directory is available as a CD-ROM or can be purchased online at www.citizen.org/hrg/healthcare/articles .cfm? ID=7383 or by telephone at 202-588-1000.

A Web site useful for caregivers and building your support

group can be found through the Family Caregiver Alliance at www.caregiver.org/caregiver/jsp/home.jsp.

International Bibliographic Information on Dietary Supplements offers a database of published, international, scientific literature on dietary supplements, including vitamins, minerals, and botanicals. They can be found at http://dietary-supplements .info.nih.gov/Health_Information/IBIDS.aspx.

A database for naturopathic physicians can be found through The American Association of Naturopathic Physicians Web site at www.naturopathic.org.

The U.S. government database and Web site for alternative medicine resources can be found at http://nccam .nih.gov.

A database for homeopathic physicians and other alternative health resources can be found through HealthWorld Online at www.healthy.net/index.asp.

A database for osteopathic physicians can be found through the American Academy of Osteopathy at www.academyof osteopathy.org.

Consumer Reports does annual comparison studies of major insurance companies, policies offered, and consumer satisfaction. This information can be found on the Internet at www.consumerreports.org/main/health/home.jsp. This same site offers good advice on how to read and understand hospital billing statements.

A good patient advocacy group is The Patient Advocate Foundation, which can be found at: www.patientadvocate .org.

Families USA, which provides a list of state agencies regulating health care and information on state managed-care laws, can be reached at 202-628-3030 or online at www.families usa.org.

A basic resource for locating hospitals is DoctorDirectory

.com, which can be found at www.doctordirectory.com/doctordirectory/hospitals/state.aspy.

U.S. News & World Report ranks the top 50 hospitals in each of seventeen specialty areas, with 205 hospitals ranked overall, based on mortality rates, available technology and services, nursing staff levels, and physician surveys. The Web site can be found at www.usnews.com.

Consumers' Checkbook Guide to Hospitals rates five hundred hospitals; mortality rates for ten common medical conditions and two types of surgery; adverse-outcome rates for seven types of surgery—all compared to national averages. They can be found at www.checkbook.org/hospital/default.cfm.

The Hospital Ratings at Health Grades Inc. provides information on hospitals and, for a fee, will provide specific rating information for requested hospitals. They can be found at www.healthgrades.com.

Prior to visiting the ER you will want to consult the American College of Emergency Physicians (ACEP), which recommends that you become familiar with the symptoms of common illnesses and injuries such as those listed in their booklet *Home Organizer for Medical Emergencies*. A free copy can be obtained by calling ACEP at 800-446-9776, or by visiting them at www.acep.org/webportal.

Myvesta.org is a nonprofit, Internet-based financial counseling and services organization, offering a free, downloadable publication, *Coping with Medical Bills*, which can be found at www.myvesta.org/pubs/pdf/medical_bills.pdf.

For more information about most pharmaceuticals, try RxList-The Internet Drug Index: www.rxlist.com.

RECOMMENDED READING

Helpful Books for People with Chronic Illness or Disease

Cousins, Norman. *Anatomy of an Illness as Perceived by the Patient: Reflections on Healing and Regeneration.* New York: W. W. Norton & Company, 2001.

Hartwell, Lori. *Chronically Happy: Joyful Living in Spite of Chronic Illness.* San Francisco: Poetic Media Press, 2002.

Helpful Books on Finding Dr. Right and Navigating the Health Care System

Levine, Evan S., M.D. *What Your Doctor Won't (Or Can't) Tell You: The Failures of American Medicine—and How to Avoid Becoming a Statistic.* New York: G. P. Putnam, 2004.

Soden, Kevin J., M.D., and Christine Dumas, D.D.S. *Special Treatment: How to Get the Same High-Quality Health Care Your Doctor Gets.* New York: Berkley Books, 2003.

Helpful Books for Hospital Stays

McClellan, Nancy, and Tasi McClellan. *Being an Advocate During Hospitalization*. Frederick, MD: PublishAmerica Book Publishing Co., 2003.

Sacco, Joseph, M.D. *Health Smart: Hospital Handbook—Get In, Get Well, Go Home*. New York: Penguin Books, 2003.

Sharon, Thomas A. *Protect Yourself in the Hospital: Insider Tips for Avoiding Hospital Mistakes for Yourself or Someone You Love*. Chicago: Contemporary Books, 2004.

Sherer, David, M.D., and Maryann Karinch. *Dr. David Sherer's Hospital Survival Guide: 100+ Ways to Make Your Hospital Stay Safe and Comfortable*. Washington, D.C.: Claren Books, 2003.

Van Kanegan, Gail, and Michael Boyette. *How to Survive Your Hospital Stay: The Complete Guide to Getting the Care You Need—And Avoiding the Problems You Don't*. New York: Fireside Books, 2003.

Helpful Books for Health Advocates and Members of Your Support Team

Capossela, Cappy, and Sheila Warnock. *Share the Care: How to Organize a Group to Care for Someone Who Is Seriously Ill*. New York: Fireside Books, 2004.

McLeod, Beth Witrogen. *Caregiving: The Spiritual Journey of Love, Loss, and Renewal*. New York: John Wiley & Sons, Inc., 2000.

Meyer, Maria M., and Paula Derr, R.N. *The Comfort of Home: An Illustrated Step-by-Step Guide for Caregivers*. Pakuranga Auckland, NZ: Care Trust Publications, 2002.

Perry, Angela, ed. *American Medical Association Guide to Home Caregiving*. New York: John Wiley & Sons, Inc., 2001.

Subjects

*Prescription for Nutri-
hing*, 2000.
*Body Tune-Up: Slow
em Running Smoothly*,
New York: Bantam

*If the Buddha Came to
Awaken Your Spirit.*

*Be Healthy: The Har-
ating.* New York: Fire-

Mind/Body

in the Heart of Pain.
, 2000.
ot, M.D. *The Healing
eventing and Treating
High Blood Pressure*,
Wiley & Sons, Inc.,

The Definitive Guide.

huna. *Alternative Med-
2001.

Pelletier, Kenneth R., M.D., and Andrew Weil, M.D. *The Best Alternative Medicine*. New York: Fireside Books, 2002.

Spencer, John W., and Joseph J. Jacobs, eds. *Complementary and Alternative Medicine: An Evidence-Based Approach*. C. V. Mosby Publishing, 2003.

Stengler, Mark, N. D. *The Natural Physicians Healing Therapies: Proven Remedies that Medical Doctors Don't Know*. Prentice Hall Press, 2004.

…ily for all of the love, …ven me throughout the … would not have been … best role model in the …my dreams, has calmed …ood health. Thanks to …nder, and Jason—who …s ago to fight for my …daily inspiration of my …la and Mariella. They …tay healthy for the rest … day of their lives.

…rst opened my eyes to … to never feel sorry for …gg, who have been lov- …t emotional support.

My agents, Jan Miller and Michael Broussard of Dupree Miller, and Associates, are wise and helpful counselors. They have encouraged me every step of the way and this book is a tribute to their support.

My researcher and literary consultant, Digby Diehl, worked tirelessly with me to make sure every important idea and medical fact were woven into this text.

Tommy Hilfiger first encouraged me to write a book. He made me feel that my message was truly important and could educate and inspire others. Tom Arnold taught me how to be disciplined in my writing, and helped me through the many health crises that seemed to never stop coming.

Many thanks to the entire professional team at Simon & Schuster/Fireside Books, including my editor, Nancy Hancock, Carolyn Reidy, Mark Gompertz, Trish Todd, and Marcia Burch.

I want to thank all of the truly caring doctors who have taken care of me, my family, and loved ones. These doctors have educated me through the years about how the medical system should work in the best-case scenario. They have inspired me and given me the most important tools to write this book: Dr. Warwick Peacock, Dr. Robert Katz, Dr. Robert Huizenga, Dr. James Sherman, Dr. George Ellison, Dr. P. K. Shaw, Dr. Mark Surrey, Dr. Peter Waldstein, Dr. Larry Platt, Dr. Joe Sugarman, Dr. Ann Peters, Dr. Ed Phillips, Dr. Jim Blechman, Dr. Arnold Klein, Dr. Stuart Gottesfeld, Dr. Jules Amer, Dr. David Bresler, Dr. Michael Odell, and Dr. Mark Purnell.

Of course, I owe a tremendous debt of gratitude to all of the doctors who participate in the Nancy Davis Center Without Walls for their continuing hard work and their ongoing efforts to help find a cure for multiple sclerosis and for being willing to embrace my nontraditional ideas of communicating and avoiding duplication. They are the true heroes who are changing the

tephen Hauser, Dr. Leslie
r. Howard Weiner, Dr.
rdette, Dr. Emmanuelle
eorge Eisenbarth, and Dr.

y helpful in the creation
, who provided many in-
d Joel Geiderman, M.D.,
ency medicine at Cedars-
sly led me through the
ered many useful ideas for

rt team, my best friends
so many health crises and
cines—their compassion,
er, Debbie Lustig, Pam
es, Tawny Sanders, Jamie
n.

, and Maureen Grauman,
rganization of the RACE
ould concentrate on this
, was accurate and prompt
er.

ver loyal supporters of my
ed so much of what this
er, Tommy Hilfiger, Tom
bbie Patillo, Natalie Cole,
s Najafy, Deb and Bill
Lyndi Hirsch, Tawny and
David Foster.

INDEX

ABOUT THE NANCY DAVIS FOUNDATION FOR MS

To contact Nancy Davis or to learn more about her foundation, write or call her at:

> The Nancy Davis Foundation for MS
> 2121 Avenue of the Stars
> Suite 2800
> Los Angeles, CA 90067
> 310-440-4842
> 310-471-4975(fax)

or visit her on the Internet at www.erasems.org/about_nancy_bio.html

ABOUT NANCY DAVIS

Nancy Davis is the happy, healthy mother of five. She is the founder of The Center Without Walls, a national medical research foundation, a noted spokesperson on MS, and the director of the RACE to Erase MS, now in its thirteenth year, which has raised $22 million for MS research. She lives in Los Angeles with her husband, Ken Rickel, and her children—Brandon, Alexander, Jason, Mariella, and Isabella.

ABOUT NANCY DAVIS

Nancy Davis is the happy, healthy mother of five. She is the founder of The Center Without Walls, a national medical research foundation, a noted spokesperson on MS, and the director of the RACE to Erase MS, now in its thirteenth year, which has raised $27 million for MS research. She lives in Los Angeles with her husband, Ken Rickel, and her children—Brandon, Alexander, Jason, Mariella, and Isabella.